ALLE · ZEIT · WACH · 1842

Progress in Pediatric Surgery

Volume 18

Gastro-esophageal Reflux in Childhood
Problems of Splenic Surgery in Childhood

Volume Editor
P. Wurnig, Vienna

With the Cooperation of
I. Klos, Graz

With 75 Figures

Springer-Verlag Berlin Heidelberg New York Tokyo

Primarius Professor Dr. Peter Wurnig
Chirurgische Abteilung des
Mautner Markhof'schen Kinderspitals
der Stadt Wien
Baumgasse 75, A-1030 Wien/Austria

Dr. Ingrid Klos
Universitätsklinik für
Kinderchirurgie
Heinrichstraße 31, A-8010 Graz/Austria

Volumes 1–17 of this series were published by Urban & Schwarzenberg, Baltimore–Munich

ISBN-13: 978-3-642-70278-5 e-ISBN-13: 978-3-642-70276-1
DOI: 10.1007/978-3-642-70276-1

Library of Congress Cataloging in Publication Data. Main entry under title: Gastro-esophageal reflux in children; Problems of splenic surgery in childhood. (Progress in pediatric surgery; v. 18) Includes index. 1. Gastro-esophageal reflux in children. 2. Splenectomy in children—Complications and sequelae. I. Wurnig, Peter. II. Klos, I. III. Title: Gastro-esophageal reflux in childhood. IV. Title: Problems of splenic surgery in childhood. V. Series. [DNLM: 1. Gastroesophageal Reflux—in infancy & childhood. 2. Splenectomy—in infancy & childhood. 3. Splenic Diseases—in infancy & childhood. W1 PR677KA v. 18 / WI 250 G257] [RD137.A1P7 vol. 18] 617'98 s 85-2797 [RJ456.G33] [617'.548] ISBN-13: 978-3-642-70278-5 (U.S.)

2123/3130-543210

Foreword

In 1968 the first contacts were arranged with the publishing house of Urban & Schwarzenberg concerning the establishment of a periodical to be produced in English with the aim of publishing important scientific work in pediatric surgery and related disciplines. I thought especially of certain excellent inaugural dissertations and theses. When Urban & Schwarzenberg promised to start such a series, I recruited Peter Rickham, then in Liverpool and now in Zürich, and Jean Prévot of Nancy as executive editors. We chose the title *Progress in Pediatric Surgery – Fortschritte der Kinderchirurgie – Acquisitions en Chirurgie Enfantile* as the name of our new series. The first volume was published in 1970, followed by another 16 volumes during the next 14 years. At the suggestion of Michael Urban, we turned from the publication of long papers to theme-based volumes, which proved to be extraordinarily useful. Mr. Urban, the head of Urban & Schwarzenberg, told us in 1982 that his firm could no longer look after *Progress in Pediatric Surgery*. With the agreement of Mr. Urban, we had to look for another publisher and found Springer-Verlag, who agreed to continue publishing *Progress in Pediatric Surgery* in the approved lay-out. We cordially thank Dietrich Götze of Springer-Verlag for his helpful support. This volume (No. 18) is the first of *Progress in Pediatric Surgery* to appear under the guidance of Springer-Verlag.

We want to express our thanks to Mr. Urban and Dr. Müller of Urban & Schwarzenberg for all of their help with *Progress in Pediatric Surgery* for 14 years. Furthermore, we want to express our thanks to Springer-Verlag and especially to Professor Götze for taking over the publication of our pediatric surgical series.

Professor Rickham retired from active executive editorship as of last year. However, he will be of further help to us as senior editor of *Progress in Pediatric Surgery*. We are pleased to have Urs Stauffer of Zürich and Lewis Spitz of London as new executive editors as well as Thomas Angerpointner of Munich as assistant editor. It is our aim to publish two or three pediatric surgical theme-based volumes every 2 years.

On behalf of the editors

Waldemar Ch. Hecker, Munich

Preface

The themes of gastroesophageal reflux and problems of splenic surgery were selected because the operative treatment of gastroesophageal reflux has been put on a completely new basis due to more recently developed methods of examination, such as pH monitoring and esophagomanometry. For many years it has been known that the effects of gastroesophageal reflux vary widely. Everything is possible, from harmless changes that heal spontaneously to Barrett's syndrome, where fatal complications and malignant degenerations have been observed. To bring clarity to the subject the attempt has been made to discuss the problems thoroughly. A similary weighty problem has become evident in recent years: following splenectomies there is a disposition to develop so-called overwhelming postsplenectomy infection. Things have become uncertain here, as well. Viewpoints must be revised and new methods found.

In addition to using the known statistics and surveys from abroad, we have tried to clarify the situation in our own area with the help of collected statistics, which are discussed by the contributing authors. We hope in this way to be able to indicate a significant direction for future work.

PETER WURNIG, Vienna

Contents

Part I: Gastroesophageal Reflux in Childhood

Part II: Problems of Splenic Surgery in Childhood

List of Contributors

ANGERPOINTNER, T. A., Dr., Kinderchirurgische Klinik der Universitätskinderklinik im Dr. von Haunerschen Kinderspital, Lindwurmstraße 4, D-8000 München 2

AUER, G., Dr., Abteilung für Kinderchirurgie der I. Universitätsklinik für Chirurgie, Anichstraße 35, A-6020 Innsbruck

BERGER, D., Dozent Dr., Service de chirurgie pediatrique du Centre Hospitalier Universitaire Vaudois, CH-1011 Lausanne

BERNHARD, U. A., Dr., Abteilung für Gastroenterologie der Universitäts-Kinderklinik, Steinwiesstraße 75, CH-8032 Zürich

BETTEX, M., Prof. Dr., Kinderchirurgische Klinik, Universität Bern, Inselspital, Freiburgstraße 15, CH-3010 Bern

BISCHOF-DELALOYE, A., Dr., Service de chirurgie pediatrique du Centre Hospitalier Universitaire Vaudois, CH-1011 Lausanne

BRANDEIS, W. E., Prof. Dr., Kinderchirurgische Abteilung des Chirurgischen Zentrums der Universität Heidelberg, Im Neuenheimer Feld 110, D-6900 Heidelberg

DICKERHOFF, R., Dr., Kinderchirurgische Klinik der Universitätskinderklinik im Dr. von Haunerschen Kinderspital, Lindwurmstraße 4, D-8000 München 2

EHRLICH, P., Dr., Abteilung für Kinderchirurgie der I. Universitätsklinik für Chirurgie, Anichstraße 35, A-6020 Innsbruck

EIBL, Martha, Prof. Dr., Institut für Immunologie der Universität Wien, Borschkegasse 8a, A-1090 Wien

ENGER, E., Dozent Dr., Rikshospitalet, Kirurgisk Storavdeling, Piledstredet 32, 0027 Oslo 1, Norwegen

ERBELDING, K.-P., Dr., Kinderchirurgische Klinik der Universitätskinderklinik im Dr. von Haunerschen Kinderspital, Lindwurmstraße 4, D-8000 München 2

ERNSTBRUNNER, T., Dr., Mautner Markhof'sches Kinderspital der Stadt Wien, Baumgasse 75, A-1030 Wien

FASCHING, M., Dr., Universitätsklinik für Kinderchirurgie, Heinrichstraße 31, A-8010 Graz

FELDMANN, M., Dr., Chirurgische Klinik der Städtischen Krankenanstalten Winterberg, D-6600 Saarbrücken

FOTTER, R., Universitätsdozent Dr., Universitätsklinik für Radiologie, Auenbruggerplatz 9, A-8036 Graz

GASS, R., Dr., Kinderchirurgische Klinik, Universität Bern, Inselspital, Freiburgstraße 15, CH-3010 Bern

GDANIETZ, K., Prof. Dr., Kinderchirurgische Klinik im Städtischen Klinikum Berlin-Buch, Karowerstraße 11, DDR-1115 Berlin-Buch

GHARIB, M., Dozent Dr., Kinderchirurgische Klinik im Städtischen Kinderkrankenhaus, Amsterdamerstraße 59, D-5000 Köln 60

GHERARDINI, R., Dr., II. Chirurgische Universitätsklinik Wien, Spitalgasse 23, A-1090 Wien

GOLLMITZER, W., Dr., Kinderchirurgische Klinik der Universitätskinderklinik im Dr. von Haunerschen Kinderspital, Lindwurmstraße 4, D-8000 München 2

GUGGENBICHLER, J. P., Dozent Dr., Universitäts-Kinderklinik, Anichstraße 35, A-6020 Innsbruck

HAAS, R., Dr., Kinderchirurgische Klinik der Universitätskinderklinik im Dr. von Haunerschen Kinderspital, Lindwurmstraße 4, D-8000 München 2

HAIDMAYER, R., Dr., Physiologisches Institut der Karl Franzens-Universität, Harrachgasse 21, A-8010 Graz

HECKER, W. Ch., Prof. Dr., Kinderchirurgische Klinik der Universitätskinderklinik im Dr. von Haunerschen Kinderspital, Lindwurmstraße 4, D-8000 München 2

HITZIG, H. W., Prof. Dr., Universitäts-Kinderklinik Zürich, Steinwiesstraße 76, CH-8032 Zürich

HÖLLWARTH, M., Prof. Dr., Universitätsklinik für Kinderchirurgie, Heinrichstraße 31, A-8010 Graz

HOFMANN, V., Dr., Kinderchirurgische Abteilung, St. Barbara Krankenhaus, Barbarastraße 3–5, DDR-4020 Halle/Saale

HOFMANN V. KAP-HERR, S., Prof. Dr., Kinderchirurgische Universitätsklinik Mainz, Langenbeckstraße 1, D-6500 Mainz

HOLSCHNEIDER, A. M., Prof. Dr., Kinderchirurgische Klinik am Städtischen Kinderkrankenhaus Köln, Amsterdamerstraße 59, D-5000 Köln 60

JAEGER, H. D., Dr., Universitätsklinik für Kinderchirurgie, Karl-Marx-Universität Leipzig, Oststraße 21–25, DDR-7050 Leipzig

KENNER, T., Dr., Physiologisches Institut der Karl Franzens-Universität, Harrachgasse 21, A-8010 Graz

KJELLEN, G., Dr., Department of Otolaryngology, University Hospital, S-58185 Linköping

KLOTTER, J., Dr., Kinderchirurgische Universitätsklinik Mainz, Langenbeckstraße 1, D-6500 Mainz

KOCH, A., Dr., Kinderchirurgische Klinik, Universität Bern, Inselspital, Freiburgstraße 15, CH-3010 Bern

KÖNIGSWIESER, H., Dr., Mautner Markhof'sches Kinderspital der Stadt Wien, Baumgasse 75, A-1030 Wien

KOSAK, W., Dr., Prosektur der Krankenanstalt Rudolfstiftung, Juchgasse 25, A-1030 Wien

KREPLER, R., Universitätsdozent Dr., Institut für Pathologische Anatomie der Universität Wien, Spitalgasse 4, A-1090 Wien

KURZ, R., Prof. Dr., Universitäts-Kinderklinik, Auenbruggerplatz 15, A-8036 Graz

LEPELLEY, M., Dr., Children's Hospital Nancy, Allée du Morvan, F-54511 Vandoeuvre les Nancy, Cedex

LÖHRS, U., Dr., Kinderchirurgische Klinik der Universitätskinderklinik im Dr. von Haunerschen Kinderspital, Lindwurmstraße 4, D-8000 München 2

LOHR, J., Dr., Kinderchirurgische Universitätsklinik Mainz, Langenbeckstraße 1, D-6500 Mainz

MENARDI, Gesine, Dr., Abteilung für Kinderchirurgie der I. Chirurgischen Universitätsklinik, Anichstraße 35, A-6020 Innsbruck

MÜLLER, Grete, Dr., Institut für medizinische Immunologie des Bereiches Medizin der Humboldt-Universität Berlin (Charité)

MUNTEAN, K., Universitätsdozent Dr., Universitäts-Kinderklinik Graz, Auenbruggerplatz 15, A-8036 Graz

NABER, M., Dr., Chirurgische Klinik der Städtischen Krankenanstalten Winterberg, D-6600 Saarbrücken

NOAK, L., Dr., Kinderchirurgische Klinik im Städtischen Klinikum Berlin-Buch, Karowerstraße 11, DDR-1115 Berlin-Buch

PFEIFFER, K.P., Dr., Physiologisches Institut der Karl Franzens-Universität, Harrachgasse 21, A-8010 Graz

PIEPER, W.M., Dozent Dr., Kinderchirurgische Universitätsklinik Mainz, Langenbeckstraße 1, D-6500 Mainz

PRÉVOT, J., Prof. Dr., Children's Hospital Nancy, Allée du Morvan, F-54511 Vandoeuvre les Nancy, Cedex

REINBERG, O., Dr., Service de chirurgie pédiatrique du Centre Hospitalier Universitaire Vaudois, CH-1011 Lausanne

ROTH, Helga, Dr., Kinderchirurgische Abteilung des Chirurgischen Zentrums der Universität Heidelberg, Im Neuenheimer Feld 110, D-6900 Heidelberg

ROULET, M., Dr., Service de chirurgie pédiatrique du Centre Hospitalier Universitaire Vaudois, CH-1011 Lausanne

SCHÄRLI, A.F., Prof. Dr., Abteilung für Kinderchirurgie des Kinderkrankenhauses Luzern, CH-6000 Luzern

SCHMITT, M., Dr., Children's Hospital Nancy, Allée du Morvan, F-54511 Vandoeuvre les Nancy, Cedex

SHMERLING, D.H., Prof. Dr., Abteilung für Gastroenterologie der Universitäts-Kinderklinik, Steinwiesstraße 75, CH-8032 Zürich

SIEMENS, F., Dr., Kinderchirurgische Klinik der Universitätskinderklinik im Dr. von Haunerschen Kinderspital, Lindwurmstraße 4, D-8000 München 2

TISCHER, W., Prof. Dr., Kinderchirurgische Klinik der Universität Greifswald, Löfflerstraße 23, DDR-2200 Greifswald

URAY, E., Dr., Universitätsklinik für Kinderchirurgie, Heinrichstraße 31, A-8010 Graz

URBAN, C., Dozent Dr., Universitäts-Kinderklinik, Auenbruggerplatz 30, A-8036 Graz

WÄHLBY, L., Dr., Department of Surgery, Kärnsjukhuset, S-54185 Skövde

WALDHERR, R., Dr., Pathologisches Institut der Universität Heidelberg, Im Neuenheimer Feld 220, D-6900 Heidelberg

WURNIG, P., Prof. Dr., Kinderchirurgische Abteilung, Mautner Markhof'sches Kinderspital, Baumgasse 75, A-1030 Wien

Physiology and Pathophysiology of the Esophagus in Childhood*

M. HÖLLWARTH and E. URAY[1]

During the past, considerable progress has been achieved regarding gastroesophageal reflux (GER) and related disturbances in childhood. This report can only present some of the results which are, in the authors' opinion, most convincing and reflect some points of personal experience, too.

Anatomy

The esophagus in the newborn child is about 10–11 cm long (Höllwarth 1979). The high-pressure zones at the proximal and distal ends of the esophagus are known as sphincters. The upper sphincter consists of striated muscles and is similar to the cricopharyngeal muscle. However, the esophagus does not show a commensurate anatomically evident sphincter system in the area of the distal high-pressure zone. Liebermann and colleagues investigated the esophagogastric junction in its natural position and tension (Liebermann-Meffert et al. 1979). A distinct zone of muscular thickening running diagonally from the lower right to the upper left side could be identified. On the side of lesser curvature, this thickening is formed by horizontal sphincter fibers of the esophagus and on the side of greater curvature by diagonal muscle fibers of the stomach. The lower esophageal sphincter (LES), therefore, originates in the junction of the two fiber systems. This muscular gastroesophageal ring lies exactly at the point of transition of the esophageal fold into the gastric fold and is clearly distal to the Z line (squamacolumnar junction) and the phrenicoesophageal membrane. The LES lies in the diaphragmatic hiatus, which is a muscular channel about 1 cm long in children, and 3–4 cm long in adults. Usually there is no intra-abdominal esophagus (Höllwarth 1979; Muller Botha 1958).

Innervation

The innervation of the esophagus reveals an extrinsic and an intrinsic system (Weisbrodt 1976). The extrinsic system, controlled by the deglutition center, is

* Supported by Grant No. 2883 from the "Fonds zur Förderung der wissenschaftlichen Forschung in Österreich".

[1] Univ.-Klinik für Kinderchirurgie, Heinrichstraße 31, A-8010 Graz/Austria

Progress in Pediatric Surgery, Vol. 18
Ed. by P. Wurnig

responsible for the function of the pharynx, the upper esophageal sphincter, and the proximal striated esophageal muscle. In the distal esophageal region, composed of smooth muscle as well as the LES, the intrinsic innervation of the plexus myentericus and plexus submucosus is sufficient for normal functioning, although extrinsic influences are present, like, for example, the relaxation of the lower sphincter by stimulation of the vagus nerve. The maintenance of the resting pressure of the lower sphincter at about 15–30 mmHg is extremely complex. Stimulating as well as inhibiting influences can be recognized in almost all known receptor systems (Goyal and Rattan 1978). In addition to a definitely proven higher baseline tension of the sphincter muscle as compared with the muscle fibers of the nearby distal esophagus or stomach, tonic effects from very different neurohumoral and hormonal substances and drugs have been revealed (Castell 1978) (Tables 1 and 2).

Years ago, gastrin was considered to be of decisive physiological influence. Since then, however, this view has been largely revised because gastrin has presumably no influence on the lower esophageal sphincter under physiological con-

Table 1. Some agents producing increased LES pressure

Hormones	*Other*
Gastrin/pentagastrin	Histamine
Cerulein	Gastric alkalinization
Substance P	Metoclopramide
	Protein meal
Neurotransmitters	Prostaglandin $F_{2}\alpha$
Alpha-adrenergic agonist (norepinephrine)	Indomethacin
Cholinergic (betanechol)	Coffee
Anticholinesterase	5-Hydroxytryptamine

Table 2. Some agents producing decreased LES pressure

Hormones	*Foods*
Secretin	Fat
Cholecystokinin	Chocolate
Glucagon	Peppermint
GIP	
VIP	*Other*
	Theophylline
Neurotransmitters	Gastric acidification
Beta-adrenergic agonist	Diazepam
Alpha-adrenergic antagonist	Morphine
Dopamine	Prostaglandins E_1, E_2, A_2
Anticholinergic (atropine)	Inflammation

ditions (Dodds et al. 1981). However, pharmacological doses, as used for stimulation of the gastric acid output, cause an increase of tonus. Important among the pressure-inhibiting substances is prostaglandin E, which is released by inflammation. This fact explains why an additional decrease of pressure of the LES during esophagitis can be observed.

Deglutition

The bulbar deglutition center, activated by neural impulses from the cortex and the peripheral receptors, coordinates the regular progression of the deglutition program.

The act of swallowing occurs normally by means of a primary propulsive peristalsis over the esophagus and effects a relaxation of the LES (Dodds 1977). During propulsive peristalsis, the esophagus is shortened considerably (up to 3–4 cm) causing a distinctive upward slide of the lower esophageal sphincter into the chest (Dodds 1977). This emphasizes the difficulty in the differential diagnosis of small sliding hiatus hernias. The border between physiological and pathological conditions is fluid (see also the chapter by Fotter, Höllwarth, and Uray in this volume).

Gastroesophageal Reflux

Several factors are responsible for the inhibition of gastroesophageal reflux (GER). Extrasphincteric mechanical factors are found in the mucosal flap, in the angle of His, in the collapse of the sphincter region during inspiration, in the pinch-cock closure of the diaphragm, in the phrenoesophageal membrane, and in the mucosal adhesion at rest (Dodds et al. 1981; Edwards 1982). It is fairly certain that the squeezing action of the diaphragm is of considerable importance (Edwards 1982; Habibulla 1972; Muller Botha 1958), which can be demonstrated manometrically in some patients with hiatus hernias (Fig. 1) and a reflux-competent diaphragm. However, it is apparent, too, that the lower esophageal sphincter alone can be fully competent and major emphasis was therefore given to the closing pressure of this mechanism. Even though the sphincter pressure in patients with reflux is considerably lower than that in healthy individuals, there is a wide overlap of pressure levels. Lower levels in healthy people as well as normal pressure values in patients with reflux have been found (Edwards 1982). Therefore, not so much the mechanical pressure barrier but, in our opinion, a functional factor has to be considered as the more frequent cause of gastroesophageal reflux. This is extensively documented by the research done by Dodds and Dent (Dent et al. 1980; Dodds et al. 1982). According to their studies, spontaneous relaxation occurs several times a day in healthy persons, mainly after meals, and results in an

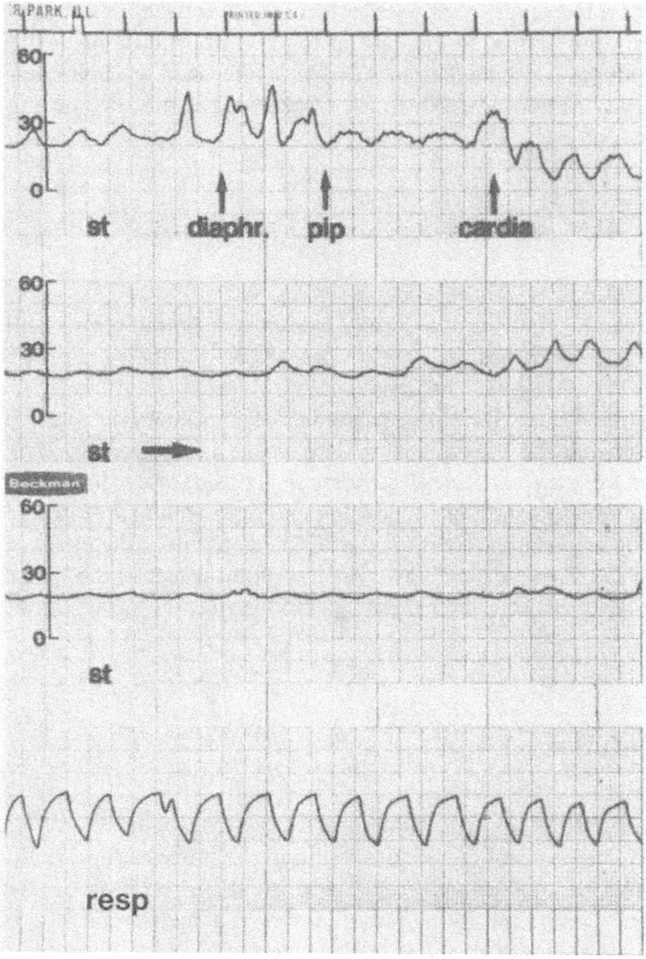

Fig. 1. Manometric tracings in a patient with hiatus hernia. The two pressure zones are clearly separated. The diaphragm *(diaphr.)* is completely pressure competent. Therefore, only intrathoracic pressure values exist in the hernia. The distance between the two pressure zones correlates with the length of the herniated stomach. *st,* stomach; *pip,* pressure inversion point; *cardia,* lower esophageal sphincter

unrecognized gastroesophageal reflux in 34% of relaxation episodes. In patients with reflux esophagitis, spontaneous relaxation occurs much more often and is connected with reflux in two-thirds of the cases. The sphincter pressure at rest can definitely remain at the normal value. Half of the remaining third of the reflux episodes are caused by an increase of the intra-abdominal pressure; the other half occurs in those phases where the resting sphincter pressure levels are under 5 mmHg during a longer period of time. Moreover, in patients with GER as well as in healthy individuals there are considerable temporary variations of the

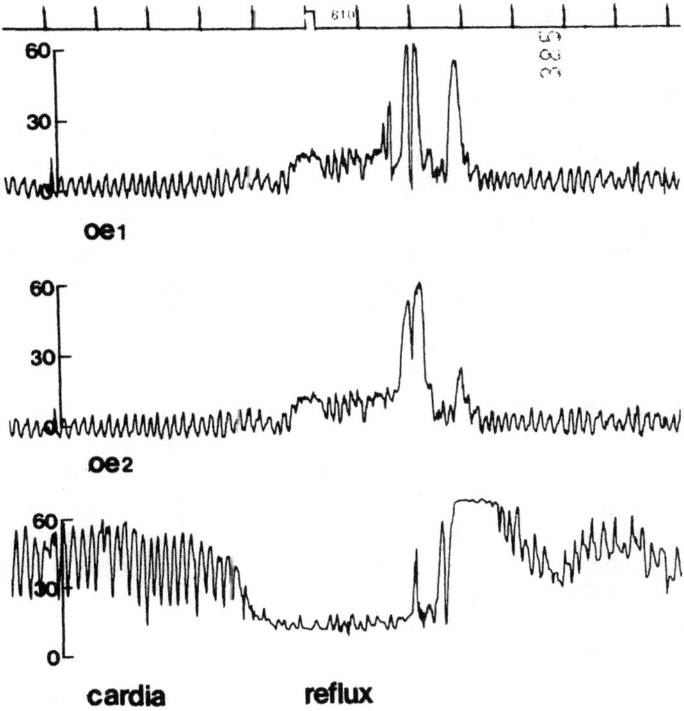

Fig. 2. The manometric GER shows the time of opening of the LES. In the esophagus it can be demonstrated by the common cavity phenomenon. The figure shows relaxation of the LES *(cardia)* and *reflux* in the upper and lower esophagus *(oe1, oe2)*

sphincter pressure values during the day. This explains why, in spite of pathological reflux, the sphincter pressure levels can be normal and reflux can also be found in healthy individuals. Investigations over a short period of time may erroneously reveal negative findings. According to our experience, pathological reflux episodes in infancy and childhood are mostly brought about by overly long relaxation phases, which can be superbly illustrated by manometric investigations (Fig. 2). In our studies, we could not demonstrate any adaptive cholinergic LES response to abdominal compression.

In infants with hypertrophic pyloric stenosis, GER usually also exists (Roviralta syndrome); GER, however, disappears spontaneously after successful treatment of the pyloric stenosis (Signer and Fridrich 1975). Whether a delay in gastric emptying is of considerable importance as a pathogenetic factor itself in infants with GER, or if it is only a part of a complex functional disturbance, is not clearly understood yet (Velasco et al. 1982; Hillemeier et al. 1981).

Development in the Child

What are the conditions in early childhood? For a long time low sphincter pressure values were postulated in the newborn. These values seemed to adjust themselves to the levels of adults in the course of a few weeks or months (Boix-Ochoa and Canals 1976; Gryboski 1965). However, the manometric equipment used lacked high-pressure pumps and the constant perfusion was technically inadequate. In contrast, our own studies using improved techniques showed that newborns already had normal sphincter pressure values which are comparable with those found in adults (Höllwarth 1979, 1980). Only the values of patients with gastroesophageal reflux were partly lower.

Newborns in the first month of life have a definitely poorer propulsive peristalsis. This means that until the 10th day only about 60% of induced swallows are followed by proper propulsive contractions. Throughout the 1st month the rate increases to 80%, which is probably a normal value (Höllwarth 1979). However, in infants with gastroesophageal reflux the disturbance of the propulsive peristalsis during swallowing is particularly noticeable and, in our opinion, it also indicates an apparent functional connection between the propulsive peristalsis of the esophageal body and the LES mechanism.

Therefore, disorders of motor coordination of the esophageal and sphincter function may be found in the healthy newborn and normally fade away by the end of the 1st month of life. Gastroesophageal reflux during the next months of life

Table 3. Three phases of the disease of gastroesophageal reflux

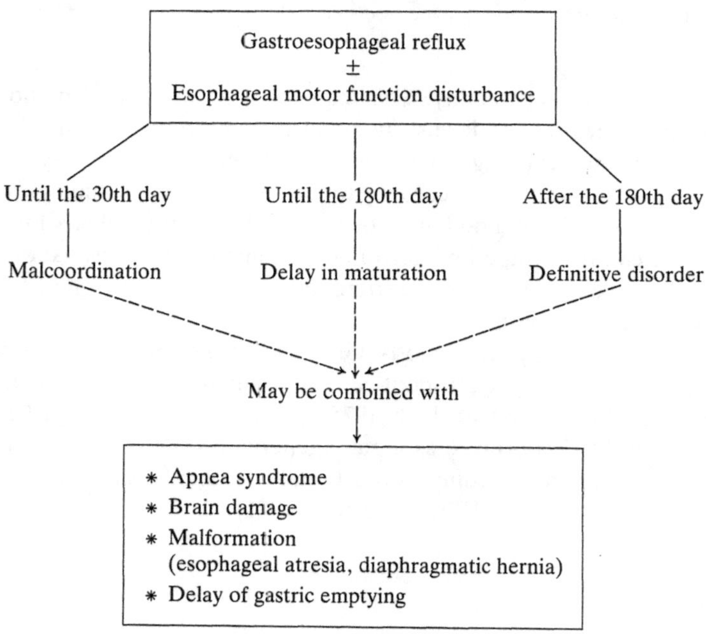

may be seen as a delay in maturation, and it usually resolves spontaneously during the first 6–9 months. A gastroesophageal reflux lasting more than 6–9 months is to be considered definitively pathological, since we have never seen a spontaneous normalization of the esophageal function with disappearance of the gastroesophageal reflux after the 6th month in any patient we have tested and examined repeatedly.

Nevertheless, it is important to know that the typical clinical signs of reflux stop generally between the 6th and 12th month and thus simulate healing. This is independent of spontaneous maturation or continued existence of reflux. This experience, as well as the fact that it was possible to show a relevant history for each of the older children with persisting gastroesophageal reflux or related complications, is basic to our working hypothesis that the gastroesophageal reflux beyond the 1st year of life is always to be considered as congenital. In the "reflux disease", therefore, three phases may be differentiated (Table 3). The first phase during the 1st year of life is accompanied by more or less distinctive symptoms, mainly spitting up and vomiting; the second phase may be with or without clinical symptoms; the third phase is (again, after years) marked by the recurrence of symptoms but now usually as signs of complications, such as esophagitis and stenosis.

Clinical Findings of Gastroesophageal Reflux in the Child

Vomiting or recurrent spitting up are the primary reasons that most children are brought in for examination during the first 6 months of life. (Table 4). As mentioned above, these symptoms almost always stop during the following months, and the children appear healthy and without complaints by the end of the 1st year (Fig. 3). Only a more thorough investigation, preferably with 24-h pH monitoring, shows whether or not the dysfunction is cured in these patients (Jolley et al. 1978, 1980). In contrast, typical reflux history symptoms, such as failure to thrive, anemia, and sideropenia, are much more rarely seen.

Reflux and disorders of motor function produce different symptoms. Reflux leads to spitting up or vomiting, with the typically related symptoms; we even have observed two children with reflux who had developed rickets. Of special concern are patients with recurring respiratory infections or asthma and those with respiratory distress (Jolley et al. 1980). Vomiting, with the subsequent effect of gastric acid, can secondarily cause esophagitis with its characteristic symptoms, such as periumbilical or epigastric pain (in childhood one seldom finds retrosternal pain), dysphagia caused by stenosis, or anemia and hypochromasia. Functional motor disorders of the esophagus only lead to dysphagia and regurgitation. Rare symptoms include the Sandifer syndrome with spastic torticollis and the protein-losing syndrome with clubbed fingers (Herbst 1978). Serious complications are reflux-induced apneas, which have a considerable importance because of their relation to the sudden infant death syndrome (Herbst et al. 1979) (see also the chapter by Kurz, Höllwarth, and Fasching in this volume).

Table 4. Symptoms in gastroesophageal reflux

- GER
  - Spitting up vomiting
    - Aspiration, Recurrent airway infection, Asthma
    - Failure to thrive
    - Apneas, Respiratory distress
    - Rickets
  - Esophagitis
    - Epigastric, periumbilical } Pain
    - Anemia, Sideropenia
    - Crying in the night
    - Stenosis, Dysphagia
    - Brachyesophagus
    - Endobrachyesophagus

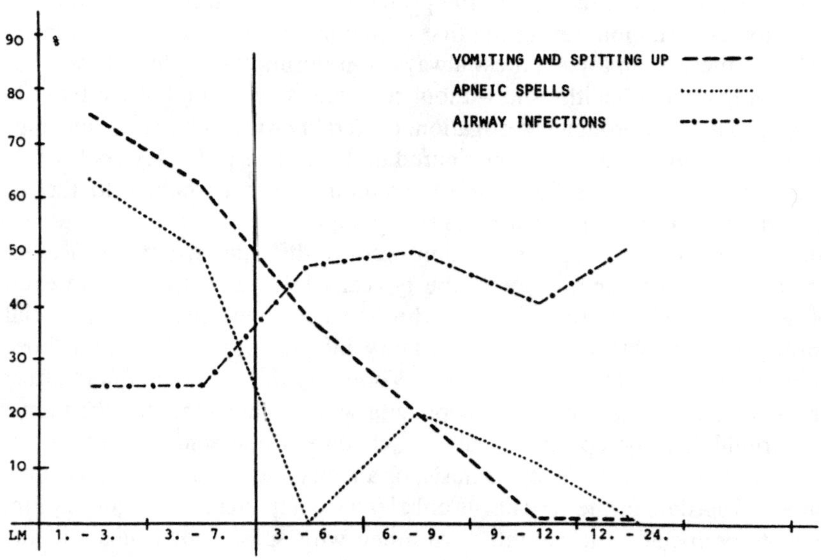

Fig. 3. Symptoms of GER, such as vomiting and spitting up as well as apneic spells, disappear until the end of the 1st year. This is independent of the spontaneous maturation or continued existence of reflux ($n = 32$)

Esophagitis

An important point in the consideration of the gastroesophageal reflux problem is determined by when and whereby esophagitis occurs and how long the epithelium of the esophagus can resist the aggressive influences of the refluxed material (Fig. 4). Among 100 fasting infants examined, we found pH values constantly under 4 in the first 6 months and levels constantly under 3 in the second half of the 1st year. The caustic effect of hydrogen ions is increased primarily by pepsin, which effects a change in the esophageal membrane much sooner than low pH levels alone. Alkaline reflux in childhood is, in our opinion, of no importance. Factors which hinder esophagitis are, beside the antireflux mechanism, the esophageal clearance for volume and acid and the resistance of the mucosa. Advantageous for quick esophageal clearance is the position of the body, whereby elevating the upper body accelerates expulsion of refluxed materials (Ramenofsky and Leape 1981). The reflux itself primarily leads to a secondary peristalsis, which is caused by stretching of the esophageal wall. Following swallows gradually normalize the pH values. It is almost always possible to find esophageal motor disorders in brain-damaged children (Wesley et al. 1981) and in patients with esophageal atresia (Fotter and Höllwarth 1979). Such motor disturbances naturally decidedly hinder the acid clearance, even when reflux episodes seldom occur.

After all, the resistance of the esophageal squamous epithelium to caustic influences is still much lower than that of the cylindrical epithelium in the region of the cardia. Acids and pepsin destroy the intercellular junctions. In the early stage of inflammation, only the surface epithelial cells are affected; the epithelial layer itself remains intact through an increased cell turnover, which can be shown histologically by the broadened basal cell layer and the relatively elongated papillae (Ismail Beigi et al. 1970). Leukocytes and round cells appear only when the inflammation advances; erosions and ulceration follow (Savary and Monnier 1980).

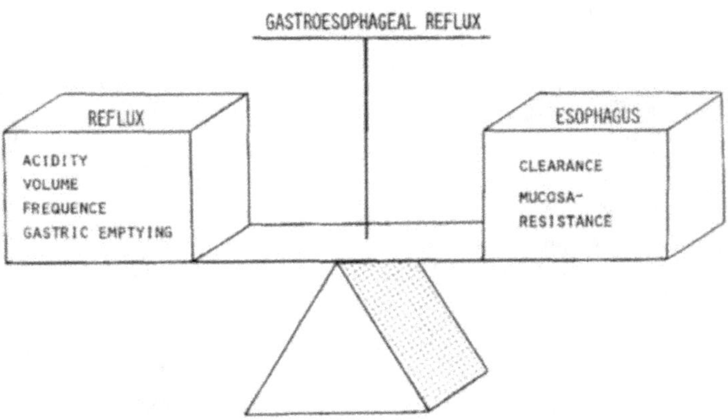

Fig. 4. The development of esophagitis in patients with GER depends on the balance between aggressive and defensive mechanisms

Brachyesophagus and Endobrachyesophagus

One of the serious complications of reflux disease, secondary brachyesophagus, is brought on by the shrinkage of the length of the organ, which is caused by inflammation. The most serious complication (especially in childhood), however, is the endobrachyesophagus, in which the squamous epithelium is destroyed by acid and replaced by the cylindrical epithelium of the cardia (Fig. 5). The significance of the endobrachyesophagus is that the metaplastic cylindrical epithelium now is not replaced by the normal squamous epithelium, even after successful antireflux surgery. Based on the adenocarcinoma rate of 10%, it must be considered as a precancerous stage (Philippe et al. 1982; Rossetti and Barone 1979). Whether or not there is a congenital brachyesophagus is highly questionable. Only evidence of an arterial blood supply of the hiatus hernia by branches of the thoracic artery could prove this beyond a doubt (Rossetti and Barone 1979). Not only the competence of the diaphragmatic pinch-cock and the esophageal sphincter but also the length of the herniated stomach, based on the distance between the two pressure zones, can be checked manometrically (Fig. 1).

The fact that in some patients the diaphragmatic esophageal hiatus constitutes a perfect pressure barrier indicates its importance as an additional antireflux

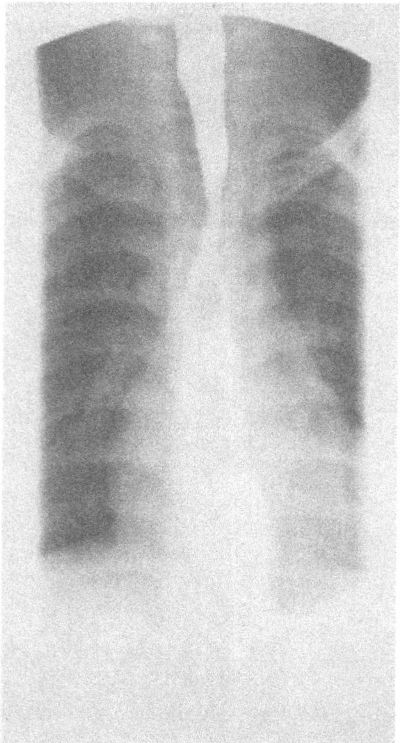

Fig. 5. A 7-year-old boy with endobrachyesophagus as well as stenosis and Barrett's ulcer. The histologic specimen showed cylindrical epithelium below the stenosis

mechanism. On the other hand, the lower high-pressure zone positioned in the thorax can also be fully reflux competent.

Conclusion

Knowledge of the functional disturbances of the esophagus in the 1st year of life – GER with the typical complications and the relationship of GER to the sudden infant death syndrome – is of considerable importance for clinicians. We are getting more and more information about "simple spitting up" but a lot of studies are necessary in the future to bring the different results into focus.

Summary

Gastroesophageal reflux (GER) is the most important disorder of the esophagus and the lower esophageal sphincter (LES) in early childhood. Functional disturbances with inadequate relaxation of the LES have to be considered as pathogenetic factors. In the 1st month many newborns have some disorder of motor coordination of the esophagus. After that time, persisting GER may be seen as a delay in maturation, which fades away by the end of the first half year. GER after 6–9 months is to be considered as a definitively pathological condition that will not spontaneously normalize. Nevertheless, it is important to realize that the typical clinical signs of reflux stop generally between the 6th and 12th month, and so simulate healing independent of whether spontaneous maturation occurs or there is continued existence of reflux. Reflux-induced apneic spells are severe complications of this esophageal disorder in the 1st year of life.

Esophagitis, usually a late complication, occurs when the aggressive factors win their fight against clearance and mucosal resistance of the esophagus. Brachyesophagus and endobrachyesophagus are severe late complications.

Résumé

Le reflux gastro-œsophagien est la plus importante perturbation fonctionnelle de l'œsophage et du sphincter œsophagien inférieur chez le jeune enfant. Les troubles fonctionnels avec relaxation inadéquate du sphincter œsophagien inférieur doivent être considérés comme des facteurs pathogéniques. Durant les premiers mois, de nombreux nouveaux nés présentent des troubles de la coordination motrice de l'œsophage. Par la suite, un reflux gastro-oesophagien peut être considéré comme un signe de maturation retardée qui disparait vers l'âge de 6 mois. Par contre, un reflux gastro-œsophagien persistant entre 6 et 9 mois, sans signe de normalisation spontanée, est un facteur pathologique définitif. Dans ce contexte, il ne faut pas oublier que les symptômes cliniques tendent à disparaître entre 6 et 9 mois, donnant l'illusion d'une guérison et il faut alors redoubler d'attention.

Dans la première année de la vie, les crises d'apnée induites par le reflux constituent la complication la plus grave de ce trouble œsophagien. L'œsophagite, habituellement une complication tardive, survient lorque les facteurs agressifs l'emportent sur les mécanismes de nettoyage spontané et sur la résistance de la muqueuse œsophagienne. Brachyœsophage et endobrachyœsophage sont de graves complications tardives.

Zusammenfassung

Der gastroösophageale Reflux (GER) ist die wichtigste Störung im Bereich des Ösophagus und des unteren Ösophagussphinkters (LES) im frühen Kindesalter. Funktionelle Störungen mit inadäquaten Relaxationen des LES müssen als pathogenetische Faktoren betrachtet werden. Im 1. Monat zeigen viele Neugeborene Störungen der motorischen Koordination des Ösophagus. Danach kann ein persistierender GER noch als Reifungsverzögerung angesehen werden, die bis zum Ende des ersten halben Jahres verschwindet. GER ohne spontane Normalisierung nach 6–9 Monaten muß als definitiv pathologisch angesehen werden. Dennoch ist es wichtig zu wissen, daß die typischen klinischen Refluxsymptome zwischen dem 6. und 11. Monat aufhören und somit eine Heilung vortäuschen, gleichgültig ob spontane Reifung eingetreten ist oder der Reflux weiterbesteht. Refluxinduzierte Apnoeen sind ernste Komplikationen dieser ösophagealen Störung im 1. Lebensjahr.

Eine Ösophagitis, gewöhnlich eine Spätkomplikation, tritt dann auf, wenn die aggressiven Faktoren über die Reinigungsmechanismen und die Resistenz der Ösophagusmukosa die Oberhand gewinnen. Brachyösophagus und Endobrachyösophagus sind schwere Spätkomplikationen.

References

Boix-Ochoa J, Canals J (1976) Maturation of the lower esophagus. J Ped Surg 11:749–756

Castell CDO (1978) Medical measures that influence the gastroesophageal junction. Southern Med J 71:26–28

Dent J, Dodds WJ, Friedman RH, et al (1980) A new tale on sphincter and reflux. Gastroenterology 79:397–398

Dodds WJ (1977) Current concepts of esophageal motor function: clinical implications for radiology. Am J Roentgenol 128:549–561

Dodds WJ, Hogan WJ, Helm JF, Dent J (1981) Pathogenesis of reflux esophagitis. Gastroenterology 81:376–394

Dodds WJ, Dent J, Hogan WJ, Helm JF, Hauser R, Patel GK, Egide MS (1982) Mechanisms of gastroesophageal reflux in patients with reflux esophagitis. N Engl J Med 307:1547–1552

Edwards DAW (1982) The anti-reflux mechanism, its disorders and their consequences. Clin Gastroenterol 11:479–496

Fotter R, Höllwarth M (1979) Röntgenkinematographische Studien an Kindern mit operierter Ösophagusatresie. Röntgenblätter 32:416–419

Goyal RK, Rattan S (1978) Neurohumoral, hormonal, and drug receptors for the lower esophageal sphincter. Gastroenterology 74:598–619

Gryboski JD (1965) The swallowing mechanism of the neonate. I. Esophageal and gastric motility. Pediatrics 35:443–452

Habibulla KS (1972) The diaphragm as an anti-reflux barrier. Thorax 27:692–702

Herbst JJ (1978) Clinical aspects: rumination and other unusual presentations of GER. In: Gastroesophageal reflux. Report of the 76th Ross conference on pediatric research 1978. Ross Laboratories, Columbus, Ohio

Herbst JJ, Minton SD, Book LS (1979) Gastroesophageal reflux causing respiratory distress and apnea in newborn infants. J Pediatr 95:763–768

Hillemeier AC, Lange R, McCallum R, Seashore J, Gryboski J (1981) Delayed gastric emptying in infants with gastroesophageal reflux. J Pediatr 98:190–193

Höllwarth M (1979) Die Entwicklung der Speiseröhrenfunktion bei Neugeborenen – eine manometrische Studie. Z Kinderchir 27:201–215

Höllwarth M (1980) Ösophagus-manometrische Diagnostik. Fortschr Med 98:712–713

Ismail Beigi F, Horten P, Pope C (1970) Histological consequences of gastroesophageal reflux in man. Gastroenterology 58:163–174

Jolley SG, Johnson DG, Herbst JJ, Pena RA, Garnier R (1978) An assessment of gastroesophageal reflux in children by extended pH monitoring of the distal esophagus. Surgery 84:16–24

Jolley SG, Herbst JJ, Johnson DG, Matlak ME, Book LS (1980) Surgery in children with gastroesophageal reflux and respiratory symptoms. J Pediatr 96:194–198

Liebermann-Meffert D, Allgöwer M, Schmid P, Blum AL (1979) Muscular equivalent of the lower esophageal sphincter. Gastroenterology 76:31–38

Muller Botha GS (1958) The gastro-oesophageal region in infants. Arch Dis Child 33:78–94

Philippe JM, Testart J, Teniere P, Bridoux J, Menard A, Leturgie C, Desechalliers JP (1982) L'endobrachy-oesophage est une lésion précancéreuse. Acta Chir Belg 4:397–403

Ramenofsky ML, Leape L (1981) Continuous upper esophageal pH monitoring in infants and children with gastroesophageal reflux, pneumonia and apneic spells. J Pediatr Surg 16: 374–378

Rossetti M, Barone C (1979) Adenokarzinome des thorakalen Ösophagus bei Refluxkrankheit. Helv Chir Acta 46:673–675

Savary M, Monnier P (1980) Le reflux gastro-oesophagien: l'apport de l'endoscopie dans l'indication opératoire et les contrôles postopératoires. Helv Chir Acta 47:693–706

Signer E, Fridrich R (1975) Gastric emptying in newborns and young infants. Acta Paediatr Scand 64:525–530

Velasco N, Hill LD, Gannan RM, Pope CE II (1982) Gastric emptying and gastroesophageal reflux. Am J Surg 144:58–62

Weisbrodt MW (1976) Neuromuscular organization of esophageal and pharyngeal motility. Arch Intern Med 136:524–531

Wesley JR, Coran AG, Sarahan TM, Klein MD, White SJ, Arbor A (1981) The need for evaluation of gastroesophageal reflux in brain-damaged children referred for feeding gastrostomy. J Pediatr Surg 16:866–871

Correlation Between Manometric and Roentgenologic Findings of Diseases of the Esophagus in Infants and Children*

R. FOTTER[1], M. HÖLLWARTH[2], and E. URAY[2]

In 1978 we began to set up a correlation between the findings of the roentgenologic and manometric investigations of diseases of the esophagus in infants and children. Since that time, we have performed 360 esophagograms and 361 manometric investigations of the esophagus. With this combined procedure it is possible to determine the exact localization of the lower esophageal sphincter (LES) in relation to the anatomical position of the esophageal hiatus. A correlation between the predominantly manometrically defined LES and the roentgenologically detectable esophageal hiatus results in a slightly modified concept of the pathology of this complicated region.

We used both methods to analyze (a) disturbances in motor function of the esophagus, gastroesophageal reflux (GER), and (c) sliding hiatus hernia (SHH). The results of the investigations disturbances in motor function of the esophagus will not be discussed in this paper.

Gastroesophageal Reflux

The roentgenologic investigation of the esophagus in infants and children with suspected reflux symptoms is absolutely necessary for the knowledge of the morphologic situation. In addition, with an appropriate technique the esophagogram permits a simple and quick detection of GER with high sensitivity (Blumhagen and Christie 1979; Fotter and Höllwarth 1981). Because the GER is a transient event, the detection of a spontaneous GER is dependent upon the duration of the fluoroscopical observation of the cardia region. But prolonged irradiation must be avoided in pediatric radiological diagnosis. Provocative maneuvers, like manual compression of the abdomen, are not physiologic and should be avoided.

In our institution we have been performing the so-called water siphon test since 1978 (Blumhagen and Christie 1979; De Carvalho 1951; Fotter and Höllwarth 1981). This is a simple and easily performed roentgenologic method for demonstrating GER with a high degree of reliability. The mechanism of the test

* Supported by Grant No. 2883 from the "Fonds zur Förderung der wissenschaftlichen Forschung in Österreich".

[1] Univ. Doz. Dr. R. Fotter, Univ.-Klinik für Radiologie, Auenbruggerplatz 9, A-8036 Graz/Austria

[2] Univ.-Klinik für Kinderchirurgie, Heinrichstraße 31, A-8010 Graz

Progress in Pediatric Surgery, Vol. 18
Ed. by P. Wurnig

depends upon relaxation of the LES which normally occurs during swallowing. In this stage the GER is best provoked and documented. We perform the water siphon test just after the conventional esophagogram. Barium sulfate suspension is given orally, and swallowing and esophageal motility are observed. Esophageal anatomy is documented on spot radiographs. A volume sufficient to distend the stomach is administered; this volume varies from 120 to 250 ml. There is a consistent attempt to approximate the typical volume of formula given to bottle-fed babies per feeding. The patient is then brought into an upright position (the infant is burped prior to the test), in order to detect an air reflux. This can be differentiated from burping through the duration of relaxation of the LES. Then the patients is placed supine and approximately 25° right posterior oblique (RPO) on the table, so that barium fills the fundus of the stomach and covers the gastroesophageal junction. From 40 to 120 ml of tea or water is then given while the lower esophagus is observed. Reflux generally occurs abruptly just after a bolus of water enters the stomach. A positive result constitutes a column of barium filling the width of the esophagus and reaching the carina or the upper esophageal sphincter (UOS). The maximal height is documented on spot radiographs. A thin trickle of barium is not considered a positive result.

The results of the roentgenologic reflux test were compared with the manometric outcomes. For this study 28 patients were completely evaluated. Of the 17 patients with a positive manometric reflux study, none had both spontaneous reflux and a negative water siphon test. While 100% of this group had a positive water siphon test, only 59% showed spontaneous reflux. Of the 11 patients with a negative manometric reflux study, two had both spontaneous reflux and a positive water siphon test. One case was a technically unsatisfactory manometric investigation, and one could be a false negative manometry. Two cases of this group had only a positive water siphon test. These were borderline cases which would not be judged positive now, but which we left in this study. The excellent accordance of the results of the water siphon test and the manometric reflux study demonstrates the great reliability of this roentgenologic technique for the detection of the pathologic GER.

Sliding Hiatus Hernia

In this disease there are numerous different statements in the literature regarding the incidence, anatomical definition, and clinical relevance.

Anatomy of the Gastroesophageal Junction

1. The esophageal hiatus is not a slit, but a channel measuring 3–8 mm in length (Botha 1958).
2. The LES is located at the hiatus or rising a little above it (Friedland 1978).

3. The thick mucosal folds of the stomach end at or below the hiatus (Steiner and Obst 1977).
4. The angle of His is more obtuse in infants than in adults and changes with respiration.
5. The upper margin of the anatomical hiatus is located higher than the roentgenologic medial contour of the diaphragm in the anteroposterior (AP) projection. The hiatus is located higher in the midpart of the diaphragm, which is ascending ventrally, but in the AP projection it is not visible. In a slight right anterior oblique (RAO) projection, it is sometimes visible (Fig. 1).

Definition of Sliding Hiatus Hernia in Infants and Children

There are two types of hiatus hernia seen in infants and children: the tubular and the locular. The locular type is uncommon.

Diagnostic Criteria

1. The LES is totally above the esophageal hiatus (Steiner and Obst 1977) (Fig. 2).
2. Thick mucosal folds extend above the hiatus (Steiner and Obst 1977) (Fig. 3).

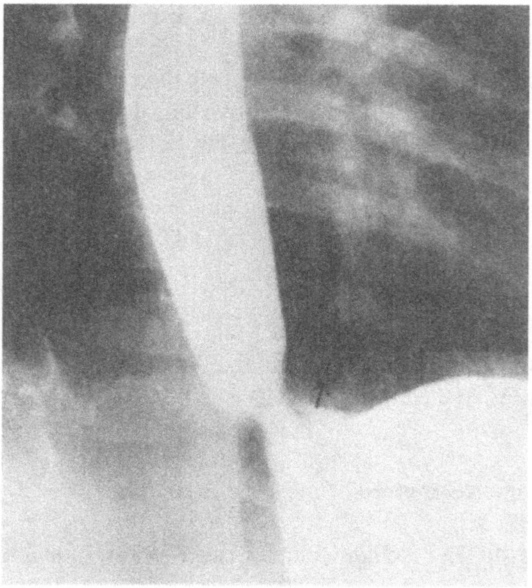

Fig. 1. Slight RAO position. Upper margin of esophageal hiatus is visible *(arrow)*

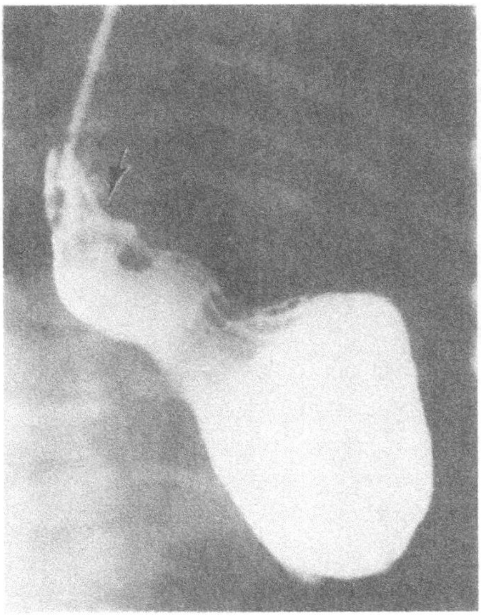

Fig. 2. Sliding hiatus hernia, tubular type. Roentgenologic LES *(arrow)* is located above the hiatus

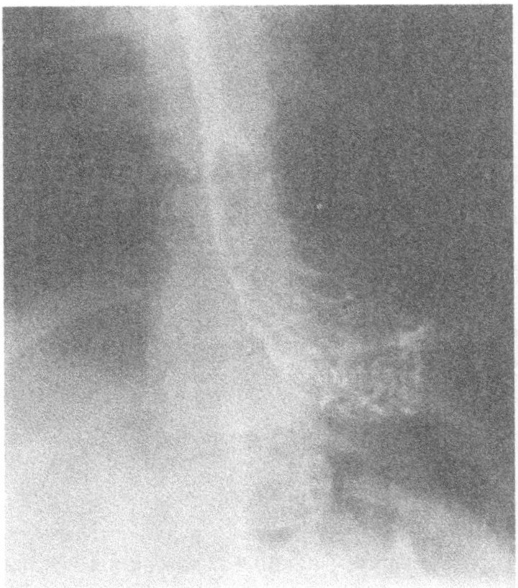

Fig. 3. Tubular type of sliding hiatus hernia. Tunnel sign. Thick mucosal folds of the stomach rising above the hiatus

3. A very wide hiatus with tunnel formation of the cardia (tunnel sign) is seen (Darling 1975). This is only reliable if combined with the criterion 1 and/or 2 (Fig. 4).
4. A noncontractible epiphrenic loculus (locular type of hiatus hernia) occurs (Fig. 5).

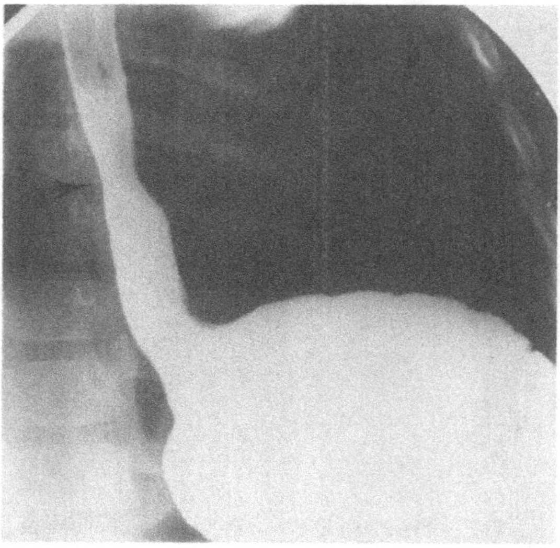

Fig. 4. Same patient as Fig. 3. Tunnel sign. Hiatus hernia. LES *(arrow)* is located above the hiatus

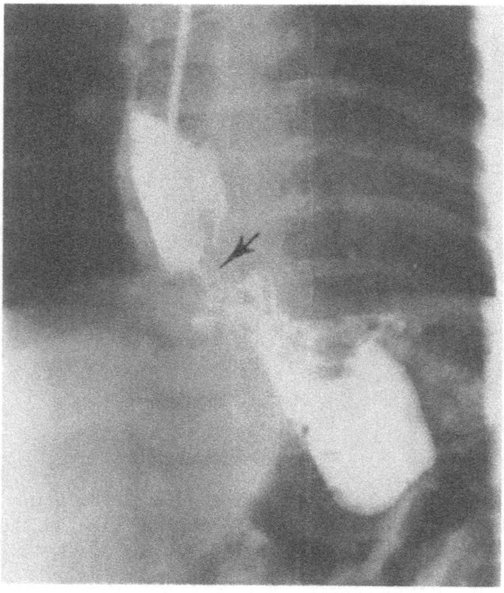

Fig. 5. Sliding hiatus hernia, locular type. Small epiphrenic loculus. LES *(arrow)* above the hiatus

Criteria Which Can Lead to a False Positive Diagnosis

1. Tunnel sign alone (without criterion 1 and/or 2) (Fig. 6).
2. Beak sign (Darling 1975) (Fig. 7).
3. Hole sign (Darling 1975) (Fig. 8).

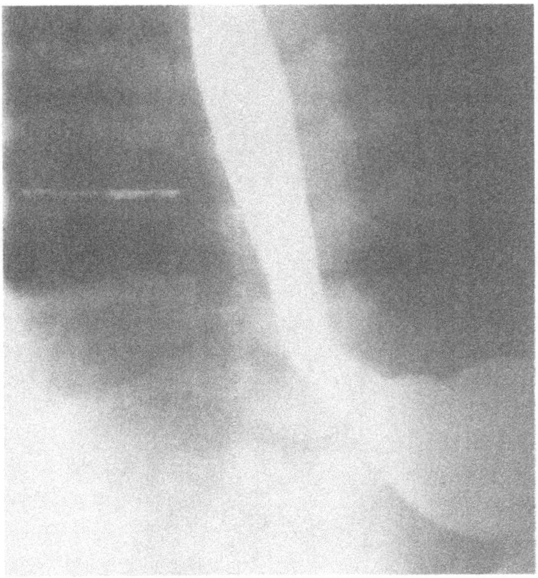

Fig. 6. Tunnel sign alone at antegrade passage; not a true hiatus hernia

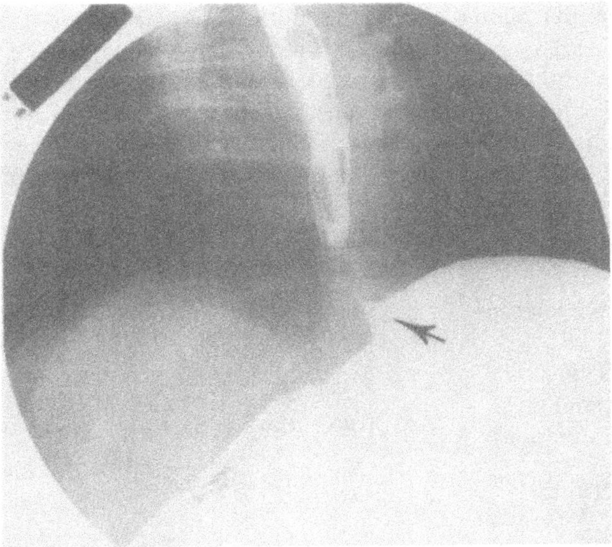

Fig. 7. Beak sign *(arrow)*

The beak sign is considered to indicate a minor degree of opening of the LES and the hiatus. More severe forms are designated as the tunnel sign and lead to an episode of GER. The hole sign alone is also only a tunnel sign during a phase of air reflux in the prone position and not a hiatus hernia.

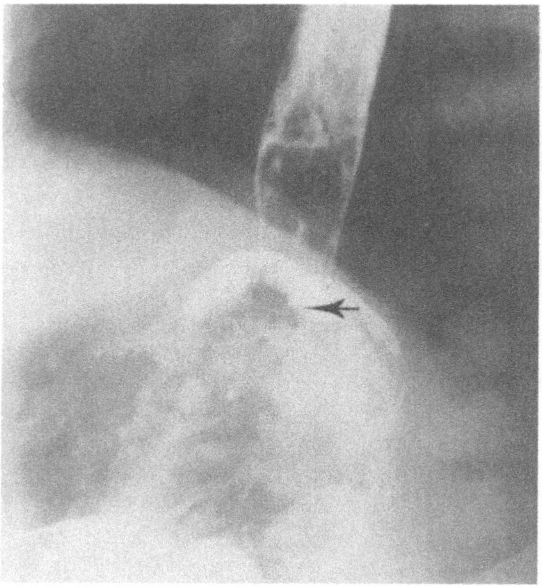

Fig. 8. Hole sign *(arrow)*

In patients who only had a tunnel sign, beak sign, or hole sign alone, we were able to exclude the presence of a hiatus hernia with simultaneous manometric and roentgenologic studies. The LES was located in the anatomical (effective) esophageal hiatus and not above. The tunnel sign represents a uniform roentgenologic symptom, but basically it is formed by different functional or organic factors. For better understanding of this probably often misinterpreted roentgenologic sign and in order to avoid false positive results regarding hiatus hernia, a definition of the different anatomical and functional forms is presented.

1. Tunnel sign with antegrade passage without GER	functional variant
2. Tunnel sign with antegrade passage and with GER 3. Tunnel sign only with GER	functional and anatomical damage (reversible) (no hiatus hernia)
4. Tunnel sign with or without GER as a hiatus hernia (see definition)	true hiatus hernia

Summary

Roentgenologic and manometric findings in diseases of the esophagus in infants and children were compared. With both procedures combined it was possible to determine the exact localization of the lower esophageal sphincter. For the demonstration of gastroesophageal reflux the roentgenologic water siphon test was used. The excellent correspondence of the results of the water siphon test with manometric findings demonstrated the reliability of this roentgenologic method for detection of reflux. In borderline cases simultaneous manometric and roentgenologic studies were also of great use for demonstration of hiatus hernia.

Résumé

Les résultats radiologiques et manométriques dans les maladies de l'œsophage chez l'enfant ont été comparés. L'utilisation des deux procédés permet de déterminer la localisation exacte du sphincter œsophagien inférieur. Le test radiologique du siphon d'eau fut utilisé pour la démonstration du reflux gastro-œsophagien. L'excellente concordance des résultats du siphon d'eau avec les études manométriques démontre la valeur de l'étude radiologique pour la détection du reflux. Dans les cas limites, l'étude manométrique et radiologique simultanée est d'un grand secours pour démontrer la hernie hiatale.

Zusammenfassung

Röntgenologische und manometrische Befunde bei Erkrankungen des Ösophagus im Säuglings- und Kindesalter wurden miteinander verglichen. Bei kombinierter Anwendung beider Methoden war eine exakte Lokalisierung des unteren Ösophagussphinkters (LES) möglich. Der Wasser-Siphon-Test wurde zur Demonstration eines gastro-ösophagealen Refluxes (GER) benutzt. Die ausgezeichnete Übereinstimmung der Befunde des Wasser-Siphon-Testes mit denen der Manometrie zeigte die große Zuverlässigkeit dieser röntgenologischen Methode. Simultane manometrische und röntgenologische Untersuchungen waren auch in der Diagnostik bei Grenzfällen von Hiatushernie von großem Nutzen.

References

Blumhagen JD, Christie DL (1979) Gastroesophageal reflux in children: evaluation of the water siphon test. Radiology 131:345–349

Botha GSM (1958) Gastroesophageal region in infants: observations on anatomy, with special reference to closing mechanism and partial thoracic stomach. Arch Dis Child 33:78–94

Darling DB (1975) Hiatal hernia and gastroesophageal reflux in infancy and childhood. Analysis of the radiologic findings. Am J Roentgenol 123:724–736

De Carvalho M (1951) Chirurgie du syndrome hiato-oesophagien (communication préalable). Arch Mal App Digest 40:280–293

Fotter R, Höllwarth M (1981) Wassersiphontest und gastrooesophagealer Reflux im Kindesalter (Korrelation mit Klinik und Oesophagusmanometrie).Fortschr Röntgenstr 135:53–56

Friedland GW (1978) Historical review of the changing concepts of lower esophageal anatomy: 430 B.C.–1977. Am J Roentgenol 131:373–388

Steiner GM, Obst D (1977) Gastroesophageal reflux, hiatus hernia and the radiologist, with special reference to children. Br J Radiol 50:164–174

Significance of Esophageal Manometry and Long-term pH Monitoring for the Evaluation of Gastroesophageal Reflux in Infancy and Childhood*

A. Koch, R. Gass, and M. Bettex[1]

Esophageal manometry and pH monitoring have found increased use in recent years for diagnosing reflux in childhood. It was, however, not taken into consideration in the evaluation of these methods that they provide different kinds of evidence. While pH monitoring directly documents gastroesophageal reflux (GER), manometry demonstrates only partial aspects of reflux prevention or relief mechanisms. Thus a direct comparison of the methods is not valid. Only the contribution of each method to the diagnosis of reflux can be the subject of discussion.

The age group mainly involved in reflux problems is certainly children in their 1st year of life. This group, however, shows dietary and behavior characteristics that must set them apart from the other phases of childhood.

In the following we shall therefore attempt to demonstrate the conclusions provided by both methods of reflux diagnosis – in infants, the larger group, by statistical methods, and in children, more sparsely represented, using characteristic examples.

Patients and Methods

Patients

According to purely clinically defined criteria, 40 infants with GER symptoms were selected at random and compared with 15 asymptomatic infants. With average ages of 4.6 and 3.1 mon ($P > 0.05$) both groups were homogenous.

The symptoms were classified into three degrees of severity (Table 1). For degrees I and II, the frequency of vomiting was the defining factor, and for degree III, it was the presence of complications due to GER. Before the special diagnosis (to be discussed later) radiological examination using a contrast passage of the esophagus and stomach was performed in all patients, endoscopy in 23 patients, and pulmonary scintigraphy in three patients with previous aspiration (Table 2).

Reflux seen radiographically was called "spontaneous" if it occurred without any manipulation, and "provoked" if it was observed during movements or attempts to drink water.

[1]Pediatric Surgical Clinic, University of Berne, Inselspital, Freiburgstr. 15, CH-3010 Berne/ Switzerland

Progress in Pediatric Surgery, Vol. 18
Ed. by P. Wurnig

Table 1. Grading of symptoms in 40 infants with GER

Grade	Definition		n
I. Slight	Moderate vomiting ($\leq 3\times$/day)		23
II. Moderate	Frequent vomiting ($> 3\times$/day)		9
III. Severe	Complications of GER		8
	– Frequent vomiting with failure to thrive >3–4 weeks	4	
	– Esophagitis/stenosis	1	
	– Documented aspiration	3	

Table 2. Previous investigations in symptomatic GER ($n = 40$)

1. Oesophagography		40
– No GER	6	
– Spontaneous GER	27	
– Provoked GER	6	
– Stenosis without GER	1	
2. Esophagoscopy		23
– Normal	21	
– Edema	1	
– Stenosis	1	
3. Pulmonary scintigraphy		3
– Negative	3	

In 34 children over 1 year (average age 6.4 years), manometrics were performed for comparison between infancy and childhood. Nine children (average age 7.2 years) underwent pH monitoring for the same comparison. The reason for these investigations were intermittent vomiting in the younger children and coliky upper abdominal pain in the school age, both of which were considered to be related to reflux noted on X-ray.

Methods

Manometry

A three-point method manometric examination was performed in the form modified by us for children using permanently perfused catheters (Koch and

Rueggeberg 1978). The resting pressure of the lower esophageal sphincter (LES) was measured as well as its competence under spontaneous intragastric pressure increase and under an increased intragastric pressure induced by manual abdominal compression. A resting pressure in the LES of >12 mmHg was regarded as normal, and a pressure of <12 mmHg as hypotonic.

If there was transmission of the fundus pressure wave into the esophagus, this was regarded as insufficiency ("common cavity phenomenon").

Long-term pH Monitoring

For the pH monitoring in the distal esophagus, a combination electrode specially constructed for infants was used (Fig. 1). It could be used in infants as young as 1 week old because of its small dimensions. Moreover, because there is no seperate reference electrode it can be used in an almost physiological way (Koch and Gass 1981).

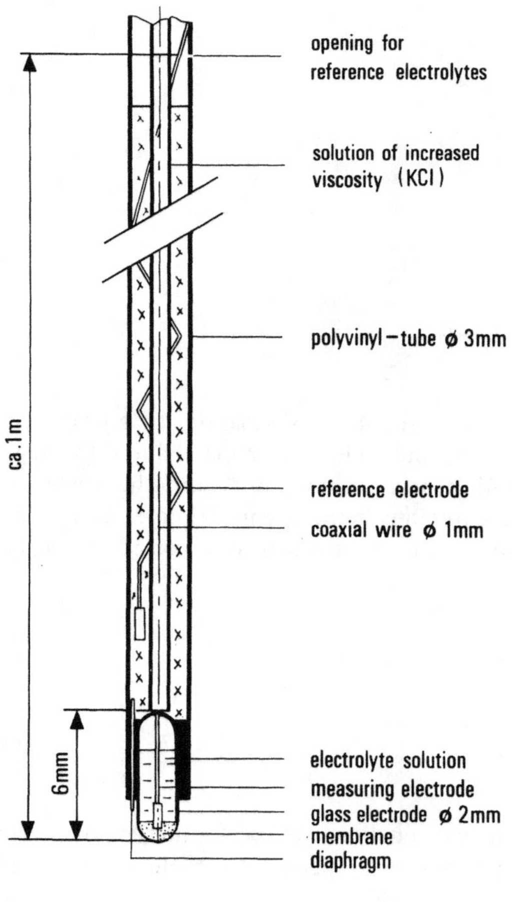

Fig. 1. Specially constructed combined pH probe for use in infants during the first weeks of life (Koch and Gass 1981)

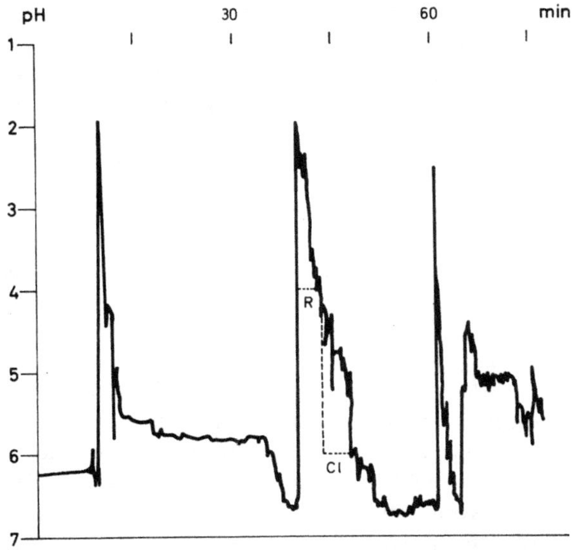

Fig. 2. Reflux time *(R)* and clearance time *(Cl)*. Reflux is indicated by a drop in pH to less than 4 for a minimum of 30 s. Clearance time is the time necessary to return pH to 6

After connection to a digital pH meter and a one-channel penwriter, the probe was placed 3 cm above the manometrically recorded cranial margin of the LES. During the 24 h of registration and continuous observation, the following indicators were recorded:

1. Vigilance (whether asleep or awake)
2. Food intake
3. Specific activities, such as crying, coughing, and regurgitation of food
4. Change of position

"Reflux" was defined as a drop in pH to less than 4 during a minimum period of 30 s. "Clearance time" was the time necessary to return pH to 6 (or 5.5, the highest value observed in one case) (Fig. 2).

Statistics

Only the pH values of the infants were analyzed statistically. Significant mean value differences between asymptomatic and symptomatic infants were obtained with the help of the unpaired *t*-test and the limits of confidence of the mean values were compared. The chosen parameters per 24 h were:

- Number of reflux episodes
- Total reflux duration
- Longest reflux episode
- Mean reflux time
- Mean clearance time of the individual episodes

The number of reflux episodes of both groups lasting ⩾5 min were compared separately.

All indicator-specific parameters with a *t*-test difference at the 5% level were tested for their separation ability by means of discriminance analysis. Auxiliary variables were established according to the marginal values of their areas of confidence.

Results

Manometry

Among the 40 infants, four instances of hypotonia and one instance of insufficiency of the LES were found. Grading the pathological results according to severity of symptoms, it was found that three hypotonic infants had low-grade symptoms, and the one high-grade symptomatic child had extremely severe cerebral palsy (Table 3). All other high-grade symptomatic patients showed normal pressure values. The only instance of insufficiency with normal sphincter pressure was found in a middle-grade symptomatic infant, also with severe cerebral palsy, induced by a hydrocephalus internus.

In the 34 children over 1 year, eight instances of hypotonia were detected, but in none of the children was there an insufficiency of the LES. In three children this result corresponded to an endoscopically verified ulcerous esophagitis. In the group between 6 and 11 years, children with hypotonia had unspecified symptoms with intermittent brief vomiting or unclear epigastric pain.

Table 3. Comparison between manometric findings and symptoms of GER in infants ($n = 40$)

Symptoms (grade)	Resting pressure of LES			Total
	Normal (>12 mmHg)	Normal but insufficient	Hypotonic (≤12 mmHg)	
I	20	–	3	23
II	8	1	–	9
III	7	–	1	8
Total	35	1	4	40

pH Monitoring

The number of reflux episodes per 24 h, differentiated as absolute and according to indicators, showed no significant difference between symptomatic and asymptomatic infants. Of the other variables examined at the 5% level, fifteen para-

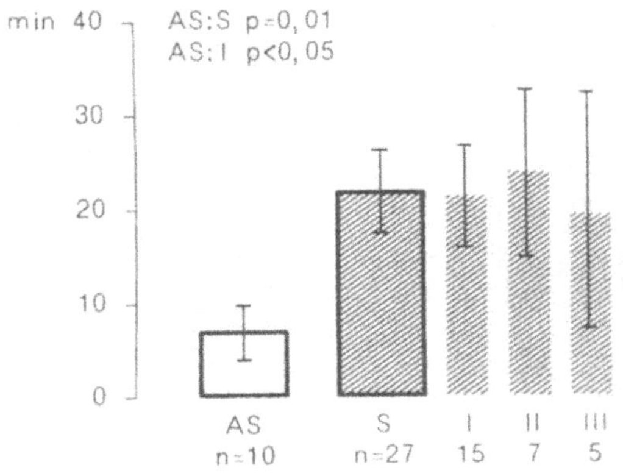

Fig. 3. Comparison of the total reflux duration/24h after the 2nd postprandial hour during sleep in asymptomatic *(AS)* and symptomatic *(S)* infants. The latter were graded into subgroups (I–III) according to the severity of symptoms ($\bar{x} \pm$ SEM)

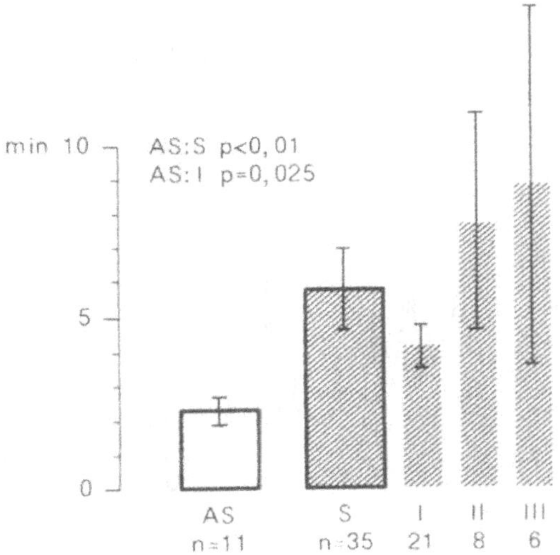

Fig. 4. Comparison of the mean reflux time/24h while crying in asymptomatic *(AS)* and symptomatic *(S)* infants ($\bar{x} \pm$ SEM)

meters could differentiate between the two groups. The discriminance analyses thus disclosed that the indicators which best distinguished between the two groups were, described with regard to the asymptomatic collective

1. The complete lack of reflux episodes and
2. The complete lack of reflux episodes outside the 2 postprandial (p.c.) hours

and with regard to the symptomatic collectives

1. The total length of reflux per 24 h $\geqslant$ 13 min aside from 2 h p.c. during sleep and
2. The mean reflux time of $\geqslant$ 3 min during crying

With the help of these four variables a sensitivity (correct assignment to symptomatic collective) of 90% and a specificity (correct assignment to asymptomatic collective) of 86.7% were reached.

By comparing the mean values of these important parameters of influence – the total length of time of reflux beyond 2h p.c. while sleeping and a medium

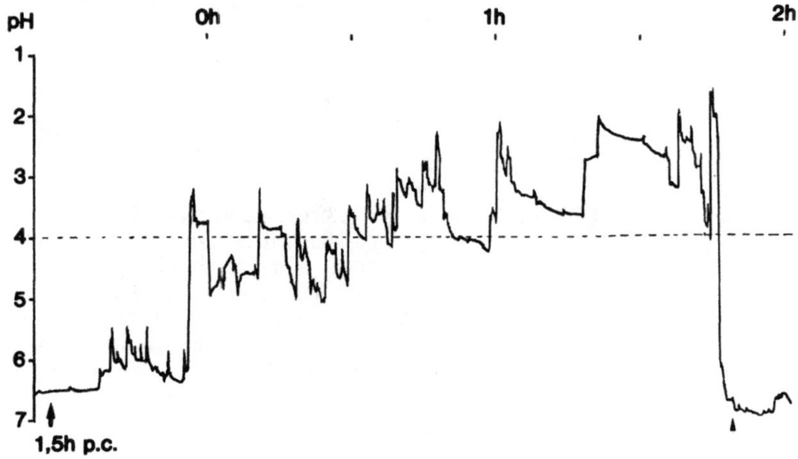

Fig. 5. Initially intermittent, then continuous reflux during restless sleep 2 h after feeding *(p.c.)* in a markedly symptomatic infant of 2 mon. ▲, next meal

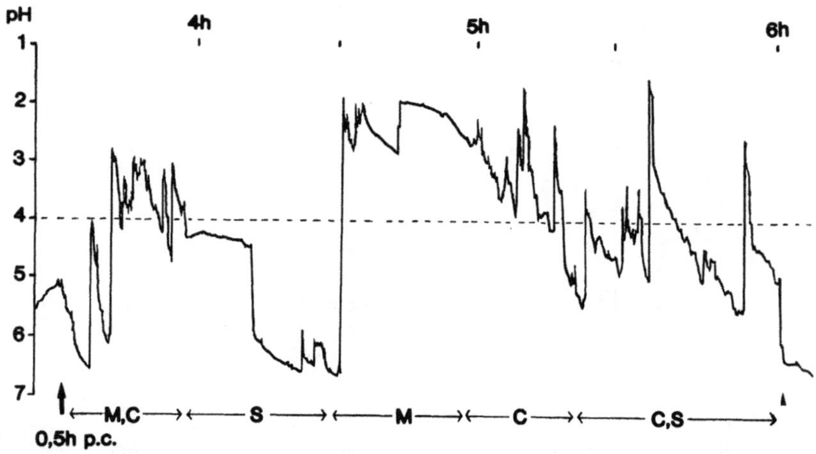

Fig. 6. Same patient as in Fig. 5 with reflux already occurring 40 min after last meal. Increased reflux during crying *(C)* and restlessness *(M)*, reduced but adequate clearance during sleep *(S)*

reflux time while crying – there were significant differences also between the asymptomatic collective and the first symptomatic subgroup (Figs. 3 and 4). Generally, the reflux became manifest after the 2-h p.c. limit (Fig. 5). The 13-min/24-h period proved to be the borderline value exceeded by the symptomatic collective on the average. In infants however who were fed on demand or who were fed more than six times per day due to poor drinking, the reflux episodes began prior to this time (Fig. 6). The more intensive the restlessness and crying, the earlier the reflux episodes with increasing acidity. The optimal dividing point for the middle reflux time during crying proved to be 3 min.

In 8 of the 2- to 11-year-old children the reflux episodes progressively were limited to the waking state with increasing age and were of a shorter average length than in infancy.

In seven children the shortness of the total and middle reflux time definitely correlated with the mild symptoms.

Discussion

This study tried to avoid the disadvantages of a collective judgment (Boix-Ochoa et al. 1980; Jolley et al. 1978) by separating the infant age group mainly affected from the other age groups differing in feeding and behavior.

For manometry, it was shown that a significant contribution to the diagnosis of reflux consists in localizing the LES and thus making the uniform placement of the pH probe possible. At the same time it gives us a first overall picture of the function of the LES and the tubular esophagus. The height of the resting pressure of the LES, contrary to the claims of earlier authors (Euler and Ament 1977), correlates in infancy only extremely rarely with the competence of the LES or the severity of the symptoms.

On the other hand, in small children hypotonia correlated better with forms of reflux complications. Therefore a hypotonic resting pressure in the case of an uncomplicated reflux was the reason for further testing and short-term control examinations.

For pH monitoring, the applied statistical methods confirmed the clinical assumption that reflux outside the 2-h period after feeding and, above all, during sleep is especially suitable to characterize the symptomatic reflux in infancy.

In contrast to the opinions of other authors (Euler and Byrne 1981), the deciding factor was not the number of reflux episodes but rather the total reflux time and/or the mean reflux time. The equation partly formed with the number of refluxes which is used by these authors to investigate the pathological reflux is called into question, as is the "scoring" largely based on the number of reflux episodes (Boix-Ochoa et al. 1980; Hill et al. 1977; Jolley et al. 1978). On the other hand, the total length of time and the average length of episodes during which the esophageal mucosa is exposed to a pH value of <4 seem to provide a more plausible basis for the calculation of risk. However, a strict association of the parameters selected by means of discriminance analysis with the severity of symptoms was not possible for any of the clinical groups or for individual patients. This could be due to the small number of middle- and high-grade symptomatic groups. But the low number of reflux complications in early infancy in general and in the patients examined here in particular seems to be decisive. This fact can be explained by the regular neutralization of the acid content of the stomach by the almost exclusively milk diet typical for this age group.

The very rare cases of inflammatory changes in this early age and their consequences indicate that there is another influence – apart from a delayed reflux clearance – which has not yet been dealt with by this method.

The observations made so far over 1–3 years on the 35 conservatively treated infants show that even highly pathological reflux values do not prohibit a rapid and definitive normalization.

In the few cases with pulmonary aspiration, either clinically diagnosed or radiologically suspected, we could not establish a correlation between reflux documented by pH monitoring and pulmonary complications despite of continuous observation. Also, in contrast to the findings of other authors (Jolley et al. 1981), there were no exceptionally frequent or long refluxes during sleep in these cases. Therefore, pH monitoring, as it is used here, cannot give causal explanations for pulmonary complications. Long-term pH monitoring has shown itself suitable, however, to deepening our knowledge of the pathophysiology of GER especially in infancy, as summarized by the following four factors:

1. Documentation of *acid* GER
2. Correlation between GER and activity/position
3. Documentation of clearance (measurement of normalization)
4. Correlation between clearance and activity/position

The conclusions we can draw from it for therapy and prognosis are limited due to the bad correlation between the original pH monitoring findings and the clinical progress.

Summary

From examinations and clinical observations of 40 infants and a varying number of children from 2 to 11 years who all had characteristic symptoms of gastroesophageal reflux (GER), an attempt was made to establish the diagnostic contribution of esophageal manometry and long-term pH monitoring.

A correlation between decreased resting pressure (≤12mmHg), or a sphincter insufficiency, and the degree of reflux symptoms was completely absent in infancy and increased only very slightly in young children.

The most influential pH monitoring parameters were reflux during sleep, beyond 2h postprandial, and during crying. These correlated most with the symptoms in infants. On the other hand, clinical developments were independent of the extent of the pH monitoring findings.

Résumé

Dans le cas de 40 nourrissons et d'un certain nombre d'enfants âgés de 2 à 11 ans, présentant tous les symptômes caractéristiques du reflux gastro-œsophagien, on a recherché l'intérêt diagnostique de la manométrie œsophagienne et du contrôle pH métrique.

Chez le nourrisson, on a constaté qu'il n'existait aucune congruence entre l'abaissement de la pression de repos (12 mm Hg) ou l'insuffisance du sphincter et l'importance des symptômes de reflux et que chez le petit enfant, il n'y avait guère plus de congruence.

Parmi les paramètres obtenus par contrôle pH métrique, il s'est avéré que les plus importants étaient les périodes de sommeil en dehors des deux heures après les repas et les périodes de cris et de pleurs, ce qui correspond fort bien aux symptômes observés. L'évolution clinique, par contre, est tout à fait indépendante des résultats du contrôle pH métrique.

Zusammenfassung

Anhand von Untersuchungen und Verlaufsbeobachtungen an 40 Säuglingen und einer unterschiedlichen Anzahl von Kindern des 2.–11. Lebensjahres, die eine für einen gastroösophagealen Reflux (GOR) charakteristische Symptomatik aufwiesen, wurde versucht, den diagnostischen Beitrag der ösophagealen Manometrie und Langzeit-pH-Metrie zu bestimmen.

Eine Übereinstimmung zwischen erniedrigtem Ruhedruck ($\leqslant 12$ mmHg) bzw. Sphinkterinsuffizienz und dem Grad der Refluxsymptomatik fehlte im Säuglingsalter vollständig und nahm im Kleinkindesalter nur geringgradig zu.

Unter den pH-metrischen Parametern erwiesen sich gerade für das Säuglingsalter der Schlaf außerhalb der postprandialen 2h und das Weinen als Einflußgrößen, die am besten mit der Symptomatik korrelierten. Hingegen gestaltete sich der klinische Verlauf unabhängig vom Ausmaß des pH-metrischen Befundes.

References

Boix-Ochoa J, Lafuente JM, Gil-Vernet JM (1980) Twenty-four-hour esophageal pH monitoring in gastroesophageal reflux. J Pediatr Surg 15:74–78

Euler AE, Ament ME (1977) Value of esophageal manometric studies in the gastroesophageal reflux of infancy. Pediatrics 59:58–61

Euler AE, Byrne WJ (1981) Twenty-four-hour esophageal intraluminal pH probe testing: a comparative analysis. Gastroenterology 80:957–961

Hill JL, Pelligrini CA, Burrington JD, Reyes HM, DeMeester TR (1977) Technique and experience with 24-hour esophageal pH monitoring in children. J Pediatr Surg 12:877–887

Jolley SG, Johnson DG, Herbst JJ, Pena RA, Garnier CR (1978) An assessment of gastroesophageal reflux in children by extended pH monitoring of the distal esophagus. Surgery 84:16–24

Jolley SG, Herbst JJ, Johnson DG, Matlak ME, Book LS (1981) Esophageal pH monitoring during sleep identifies children with respiratory symptoms from gastroesophageal reflux. Gastroenterology 80:1501–1506

Koch A, Rueggeberg J (1978) Zur Funktion des unteren Oesophagussphinkters im Säuglingsalter. Langenbecks Arch Chir [Suppl] 53–57

Koch A, Gass R (1981) Continuous 20–24-hr esophageal pH monitoring in infancy. J Pediatr Surg 16:109–113

Progress in the Diagnosis of Gastroesophageal Reflux in Childhood: 24-Hour pH Monitoring

K.-P. Erbelding, F. Siemens, and T. A. Angerpointner[1]

Introduction

For the past several years, 24-h pH monitoring has been applied in adult medicine as well as in pediatrics in the United States. This is well documented in a number of publications (De Meester and Johnson 1976; Euler and Byrne 1981; Hill et al. 1977; Johnson and De Meester 1974; Jolley et al. 1978, 1981). In Europe, however, this method has not yet come into general use. The introduction of esophageal pH monitoring in pediatric surgery was particularly influenced by Boix-Ochoa of Barcelona (1979) and Koch of Bern (personal communication, 1983). We have been using 24-h pH monitoring as a routine diagnostic method at our hospital since May 1982.

Materials and Methods

Our pH monitoring device consists of a pH probe, a pH meter, and a pen writer.

At the moment, we are using the combined pH probe 440 M 4 (manufactured by Ingold, Zurich/Frankfurt) with a diameter of 4 mm and a length of the glass probe of 20 mm. These dimensions allow transnasal positioning of the probe 2–3 cm above the lower esophageal sphincter. The exact position is controlled either by radiography, manometry, or pH monitoring, or by the combination of these methods. Radiography shows the tip of the probe at the level of the diaphragm; in manometric control, first the position of the lower esophageal sphincter (high-pressure zone) must be found, then the distance is measured, and the probe brought into place thereafter. In control by pH monitoring, the probe is first put into the stomach, which is characterized by low pH values, and then gradually withdrawn. A sharp pH increase shows the border between esophagus and stomach. Then the probe is fixed 2–3 cm above this border. An exact positioning of the probe was possible in all patients using these methods. The long probe wire (length 3 m) is connected to the pH meter (digital pH meter 646 manufactured by Knick, Berlin). The pH meter is in turn connected to a pen writer, which registers the data continuously.

[1] Dept. of Pediatric Surgery, University Children's Hospital, Lindwurmstr. 4, D-8000 Munich/F.R.G.

Progress in Pediatric Surgery, Vol. 18
Ed. by P. Wurnig

The children are normally fed immediately after positioning of the probe and setting up of the equipment. Problems caused by the probe were seen in only one patient, who had been operated for esophageal atresia. The children were not sedated. It was possible for the parents to carry the children around and play with them, since they usually tolerated the procedure well after a short period of adaptation.

The following data were obtained through pH monitoring:

1. A drop in pH below 4
2. Duration of reflux episodes
3. Frequency of reflux episodes
4. Clearance time, i.e., the time necessary to return pH to normal

According to these criteria, a pathological GER was easily diagnosed.

Results

We have used 24-h pH monitoring in 43 children since May 1982. A few examples of pH recordings in our patients may be demonstrated (Figs. 1–5).

Case 1 (Fig. 1). Three-week-old infant, operated for double jejunal atresia, no spitting-up, no vomiting. pH monitoring showed unconspicious findings. Diagnosis: NAD (no abnormality discovered).

Case 2 (Fig. 2). Three-month-old girl with relaxatio diaphragmatica and radiological signs of an upside-down stomach. Preoperative 24-h pH monitoring showed

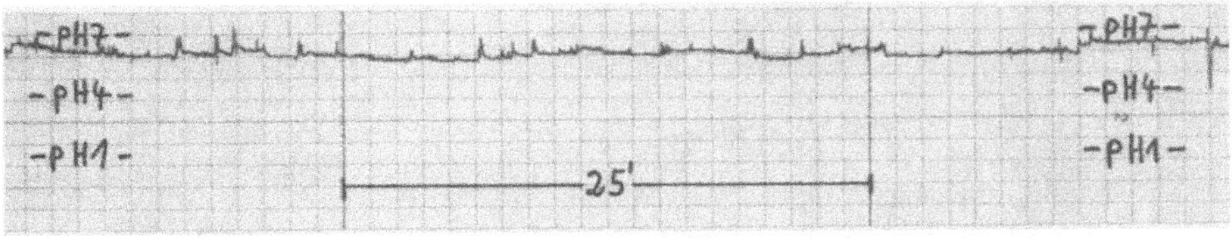

Fig. 1. Record of pH monitoring in a 3-week-old infant with normal cardia. Time in min *(horizontal line)*, pH values *(vertical line)*. Only one short reflux episode with normal clearance time *(right-hand side)*

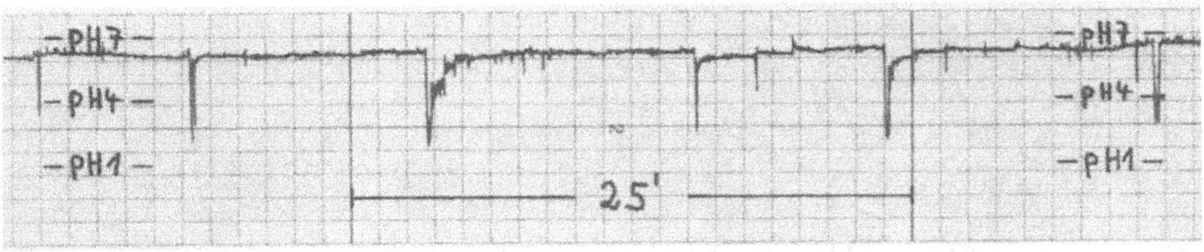

Fig. 2. Preoperative record of pH monitoring in a 3-mon-old girl with radiological evidence of an upside-down stomach. Several short reflux episodes with normal clearance time

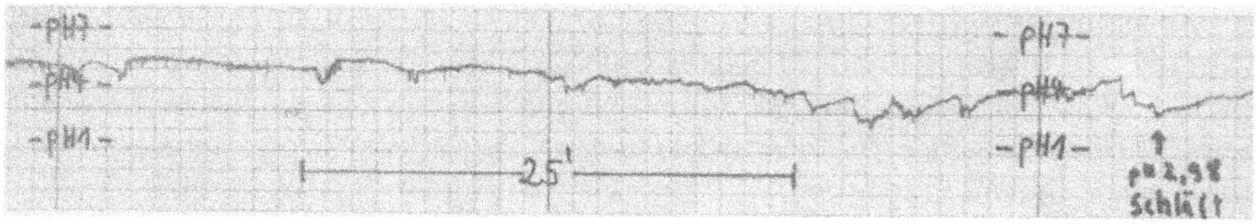

Fig. 3. Record of a 5-week-old girl with recurrent vomiting; operations for repair of myelomeningocele and for correction of hydrocephalus. Slow decrease of pH below 4; no clearance; very slow increase of pH above 4. Diagnosis of cardial insufficiency with long-standing GER

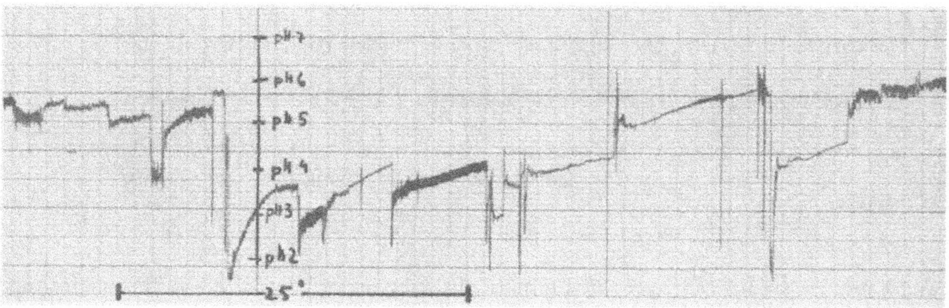

Fig. 4. Record of 2-mon-old boy with recurrent vomiting; radiological signs of severe GER; operation for repair of omphalocele. Frequent reflux episodes, delayed clearance. Diagnosis of severe cardial insufficiency with GER

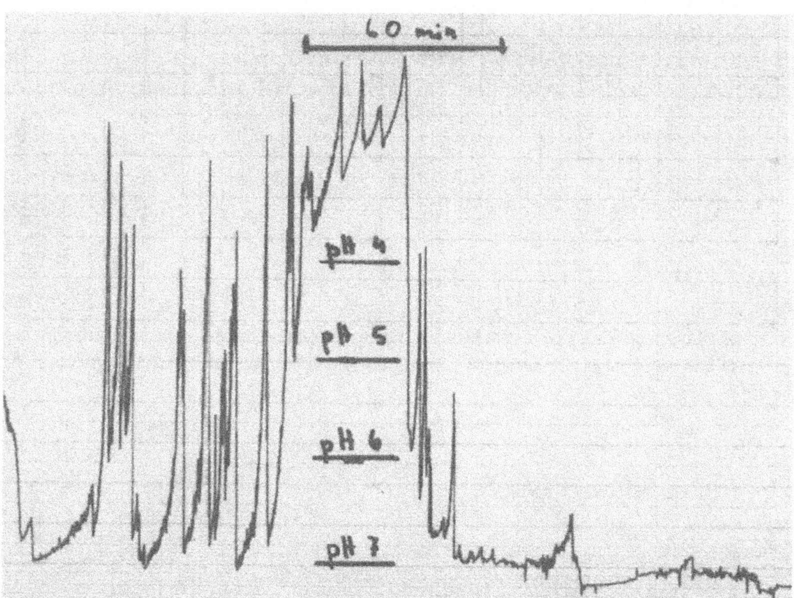

Fig. 5. Record of 5-year-old boy who had been operated on to correct an esophageal atresia (Vogt IIIb). Recurrent bronchopneumonia. No radiological evidence of GER. Frequent reflux episodes with delayed clearance. Diagnosis of severe cardial insufficiency with GER

normal conditions with only short reflux episodes and normal clearance time. Diagnosis: NAD.

Case 3 (Fig. 3). Five-week-old girl, operated for myelomeningocele and hydrocephalus, recurrent vomiting. pH monitoring revealed a steadily decreasing pH below 4, no clearance, very slow pH increase above 4. Diagnosis: cardial insufficiency with severe GER.

Case 4 (Fig. 4). Two-week-old boy, operated for omphalocele; recurrent vomiting, radiological signs of severe GER. pH monitoring showed frequent reflux-episodes with delayed clearance. Diagnosis: severe cardial insufficiency with GER.

Case 5 (Fig. 5). Five-year-old boy who had been operated for esophageal atresia (Vogt IIIb); recurrent bronchopneumonias. Radiologically no signs of GER evident; pH monitoring revealed frequent reflux episodes of longer duration. Diagnosis: cardial insufficiency with severe GER.

Discussion

Methods applied for the diagnosis of GER in adults are of considerably less use in children, since children are uncooperative and unable to express their complaints (Blum and Siewert 1981). GER was proven radiologically in only 58% of adults and 65% of children with symptoms of severe reflux and absolute indication for surgery (Hill et al. 1977). Endoscopy is also limited use in diagnosis, since 44% of the patients with clinical signs of severe GER show no change of the esophageal mucosa (De Meester and Johnson 1976). The unreliability of these methods as well as the difficulties encountered in infants and children require very time-consuming procedures and often render an exact investigation impossible.

In contrast, 24-h pH monitoring is

1. Easy to apply because (a) the children need not be sedated, (b) the positioning of the probe requires very little time, and (c) normal activities are possible after setting up of the equipment.
2. More physiological, since the function of cardia and esophagus can be measured over 24 h without maneuvers like pressure on the abdomen and instillation of an acid or a radioactive substance.
3. More reliable, since long-term evaluation is possible, the procedure is reproducible, and false-negative results can be avoided by correct application and intact equipment.

For these reasons, 24-h pH monitoring should be preferred in future for the diagnosis of GER in pediatric surgery and pediatrics if recurrent vomiting, recurrent bronchopneumonia, apneic spells of unknown origin, and near-miss sudden infant death are conditions being investigated.

Summary

Twenty-four-hour pH monitoring is a reliable and secure method for use in the diagnosis of gastroesophageal reflux (GER). Compared with other methods, this technique is well tolerated and without complications. In contrast to other techniques (cineradiography, manometry, scintiscanning, endoscopy), long-term pH monitoring is the only method to measure the dynamics in the distal esophagus under nearly physiological conditions and to register the data obtained via pen writer for any time desired. Thus, 24-h pH monitoring is the most sensitive and expressive method for the diagnosis of GER in childhood, providing more secure operative indications combined with other methods.

Résumé

Un contrôle pH métrique sur une période de 24 h est une méthode fiable, bien tolérée et ne comportant aucun risque de complications pour le diagnostique du reflux gastro-œsophagien. Contrairement à d'autres méthodes, telles que la radiologie, la manométrie, la scintigraphie et l'endoscopie, le contrôle pH métrique permet d'étudier l'œsophage dans des conditions quasi physiologiques et d'enregistrer les résultats durant n'importe quel laps de temps souhaité. C'est donc la méthode de choix pour un examen minutieux et révélateur et pour le diagnostic du reflux gastro-œsophagien chez l'enfant.

En combinaison avec les autre examens mentionnés, le contrôle pH métrique sur une période de 24 h permet de poser l'indication de l'intervention en toute connaissance de cause et sécurité.

Zusammenfassung

In der Diagnostik des gastroösophagealen Refluxes (GER) ist die 24-h-pH-Metrie eine genaue und sichere Untersuchungsmethode. Diese Methode ist im Vergleich zu anderen Untersuchungsmethoden wenig belastend und ohne nennenswerten Komplikationen. Im Gegensatz zu den anderen Methoden (Röntgen, Manometrie, Szintigraphie, Ösophagoskopie) ist die Langzeit-pH-Metrie als einzige in der Lage, die Vorgänge im distalen Ösophagus unter nahezu physiologischen Verhältnissen zu studieren und, mittels eines Schreibers, über jeden gewünschten Zeitraum festzuhalten. Die 24-h-pH-Metrie ist somit die empfindlichste und aussagekräftigste Untersuchungsmethode in der Diagnostik des gastroösophagealen Refluxes im Kindesalter. In Verbindung mit den anderen genannten Untersuchungsmethoden wird dadurch die Indikationsstellung zur Operation sicherer.

References

Blum AL, Siewert JR (1981) Refluxtherapie. Springer, Heidelberg New York

Boix-Ochoa J (1979) Report of the 76th Ross conference on pediatric research 1979. Ross Laboratories, Columbus, Ohio

DeMeester TR, Johnson LF (1976) The evaluation of objective measurements of gastroesophageal reflux and their contribution to patient management. Surg Clin North Am 56:39

Euler AR, Byrne WJ (1981) Twenty-four-hour esophageal intraluminal pH probe testing: a comparative analysis. Gastroenterology 80:957–961

Hill JL, Pellegrini CA, Burrington JD, Reyes HM, DeMeester TR (1977) Technique and experience with 24-hour esophageal pH monitoring in children. J Ped Surg 12:877–887

Johnson DG, DeMeester TR (1974) Twenty-four-hour pH monitoring of the distal esophagus. A qualitative measure of gastroesophageal reflux. Am J Gastroenterol 62:325

Jolley SG, Johnson DG, Herbst JJ, Perra A, Garnier R (1978) An assessment of gastroesophageal reflux in children by extended pH monitoring of the distal esophagus. Surgery 84:16–22

Jolley SG, Herbst JJ, Johnson DG, Matlak ME, Book LS (1981) Esophageal pH monitoring during sleep identifies children with respiratory symptoms from gastroesophageal reflux. Gastroenterology 80:1501–1506

Endoscopic Findings in Reflux Esophagitis in Childhood

H. D. JAEGER[1]

Until 1980 at our clinic all endoscopic investigations of the esophagus and stomach were done using rigid instruments. After that time, we began using a flexible gastroesophagoscope for children (Olympus GIF – P II).

The introduction of this instrument has changed our attitude concerning the way of investigation.

As the quality of information obtained by endoscopy is by far superior to that obtained by roentgenology, which had up to this point been the prevailing form of investigation of the upper intestinal tract, our checkup program has been changed to relegate roentgenologic examinations to second place.

Figure 1 summarizes all esophagoscopies performed in 1982 and shows that this procedure has also been applied during the first months of life.

Up to the age of 10 years, the endoscopies were performed under general anesthesia; in older children we tried it with sedation only, depending on how cooperative the children were. In only one child, a 12-year-old girl, did we have to give up and finish endoscopy under general anesthesia. We did not face any severe complications, even in young babies; specifically, tracheal compressions, as reported in the literature, were not seen with optimal posture of the patient and careful anesthesia.

Table 1 shows the indications for endoscopy and the rate of esophagitis. We were surprised by the fact that in spite of the high number of operations of over 3500 per year, we have found hardly any complications of reflux esophagitis recently. This is also documented by our operative rate for hiatus hernia. While during the 1960s and early 1970s we did an average of 10–12 gastropexies or

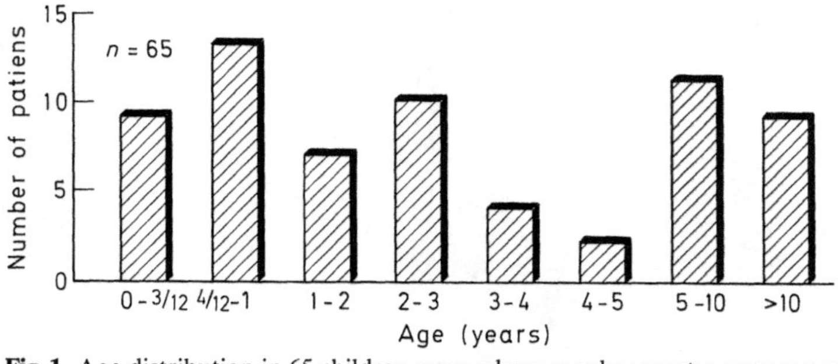

Fig. 1. Age distribution in 65 children upon whom esophagogastrocopy was performed in 1982

[1]University Clinic of Pediatric Surgery, Karl-Marx-University Leipzig, Oststr. 21–25, DDR-705 Leipzig

Progress in Pediatric Surgery, Vol. 18
Ed. by P. Wurnig

Table 1. Esophagogastroscopies performed in 1982

Indication	Number of patients	Patients with esophagitis
Esophageal varicosis	12	
Hypertrophic pyloric stenosis	11	3
Roviralta syndrome	3	2
Lye lesion	11	
Operated esophageal atresia	9	2
Gastric or duodenal ulcer	5	1
Other conditions	14	2
Total	65	10

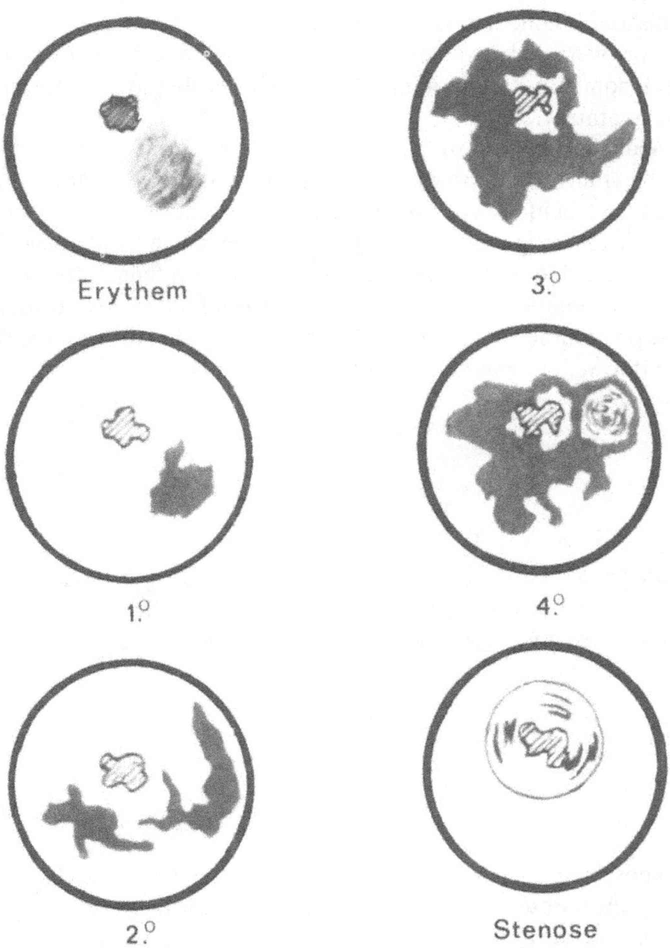

Fig. 2. Stages of reflux esophagitis, according to Savry and Miller

fundoplications yearly, we have found an indication for these operations only three times during the last 5 years.

For classification of our endoscopic findings, we use the staging rules by Sawary and Miller (Fig. 2), but we would like to add the erythema as an early phase of an inflammatory reaction, as in such cases there was always evidence of incompetence of the cardia under simultaneous manometric investigation. We are unable to report on bioptic findings yet, but we shall add this possibility in selected patients in the future. In babies suffering from pyloric stenosis and Roviralta syndrome, with esophagoscopy we found inflammatory reactions (stage 1 and 2) after prolonged disease. In three patients with Roviralta syndrome, there were two instances of stage 2 esophagitis. The majority of cases of esophagitis belonged to stages 1 and 2. We are unable to show any advanced forms of reflux esophagitis, as no such cases have turned up since colored endophotography has been at our disposal. This favorable development is apparently the result of an optimal early diagnosis by our pediatrician colleagues.

Thus, years ago we were led to abandon our previous concept of therapy under the influence of sometimes disappointing operative results, to give preference to conservative treatment.

In summary we should like to stress that for the planning of treatment, esophagoscopy has proved to be an investigation which gives us most valuable information without causing too much trouble to our little patients. It is superior to roentgenographic investigation of the esophagus in recognizing an esophagitis at stages 1 and 2. In addition it is valuable in the follow-up of all kinds of inflammatory disorders. The endoscopic evaluation of the esophageal mucosa holds a key position among the diagnostic possibilities of reflux esophagitis, which otherwise consist of manometry, pH monitoring, and mucosal biopsy.

Summary

The position of esophagoscopy as a diagnostic aid in reflux esophagitis in 65 cases is discussed. Especially since fiberscopes have come into use, the diagnosis of reflux esophagitis by endoscopy is absolutely better than with radiological procedures.

Résumé

Le rôle de l'œsophagoscopie en tant qu'aide diagnostique dans les œsophagites par reflux est discuté, après observation de 65 cas. On a pu constater que, depuis l'utilisation des fibroscopes surtout, l'endoscopie permet un diagnostic beaucoup plus exact que la radiologie et doit donc être la méthode de choix.

Zusammenfassung

Es wird über die derzeitige Stellung der Ösophagoskopie in der Diagnostik der Refluxösophagitis anhand von 65 Fällen berichtet. Besonders der Einsatz der Glasfiberendoskopie läßt eine viel exaktere Diagnostik der Refluxösophagitis zu, so daß die Endoskopie hier gegenüber der Röntgenuntersuchung vorrangig ist.

References

Becker M (1979) Gastrointestinale Endoskopie im Kindesalter: Erfahrungen mit 211 Untersuchungen. Z Kinderchir [Suppl] 27:70–76

Blum AL (1978) Die Refluxkrankheit aus internistischer Sicht. Chirurg 49:129–136

Burdelski M (1978) Endoscopy in pediatric gastroenterology. Eur J Pediatr 128:33–39

Dangel P (1979) Indikation, Technik und Gefahren der Narkose im Rahmen endoskopischer Untersuchungen bei Kindern. Z Kinderchir [Suppl] 27:14–23

Fleig W, Rüttenauer K, Belohlavek D (1979) Erfahrungen aus 2 Jahren pädiatrischer Endoskopie des oberen und unteren Verdauungstraktes. Z Kinderchir [Suppl] 27:77–80

Höpner F (1979) Kinderchirurgische Indikationen zur Endoskopie des Ösophagus. Z Kinderchir [Suppl] 27:54–58

Koch A (1980) Die Kardiainsuffizienz im Säuglings- und Kindesalter. Pädiat Fortbildk Praxis 49:32–50

Meissner F (to be published) Die Operationsindikation bei gastrooesophagealem Reflux (kardiooesophageales Syndrom)

Morphological Findings in Peptic Esophageal Stenosis with Barrett's Ulcer in Children

P. WURNIG, R. KREPLER, and W. KOSAK[1]

Today it is a well-known fact that reflux esophagitis with its serious complications of peptic stenosis (Savary and Miller 1976; Shmerling 1976; Wienbeck et al. 1976) and possibly Barrett's ulcer (Barrett 1951; Wurnig 1963) (Tables 1 and 2) often occurs in hiatus hernia in infants and children. This knowledge is supported and extended mainly by the results of pH monitoring and esophageal manometry

Table 1. Synonyms for the so-called Barrett's syndrome

1. Ulcus oesophagi (Barrett 1951)
2. Peptic esophageal stenosis (Barrett 1951)
3. Barrett's ulcer (Barrett 1951; Wienbeck et al. 1976)
4. Brachyesophagus, Endobrachyesophagus (Konrad and Rotthof 1959; Savary and Miller 1976; Wienbeck et al. 1976)
5. Brachyoesophagus congenitus (Huber 1959; Konrad and Rotthof 1959; Savary and Miller 1976; Wienbeck et al. 1976)
6. Ascending fibrosis of the esophagus (Kelly Brown 1930)
7. Peptic esophageal stenosis with marginal ulceration (Wolf et al. 1955, 1958)
8. Peptic ulcer of the esophagus with partial thoracic stomach (Stewart, Hartfall) (Wurnig 1955a)
9. Esophagus lined with gastric mucosa (Allison 1949)
10. Intrathoracic displacement of the cardia without hiatus hernia (Wurnig 1955a)

Table 2. Stages of the "short esophagus", i.e., conditions as listed in Table 1 (Wurnig 1963)

Stage	Endoscopy	Radiology	Anatomy
I	Gastroesophageal reflux, catarrhal or erosive esophagitis	Temporary spasm of the lower esophagus with shortening or hiatus hernia; "congenital brachyesophagus"	
II	Gastroesophageal reflux, erosive or ulcerous esophagitis, stenosis, infiltration of the wall of the esophagus	Permanent stenosis and shortening of the esophagus, always hiatus hernia	Flat, longitudinal ulcerations of the squamous epithelium, inflammation of the esophageal wall, and periesophagitis

[1]Mautner-Markhofsches Kinderspital der Stadt Wien, Baumgasse 75, A-1030 Vienna/Austria

Progress in Pediatric Surgery, Vol. 18
Ed. by P. Wurnig

Table 2 (continued)

Stage	Endoscopy	Radiology	Anatomy
III	Gastroesophageal reflux, severe ulcerous pseudo-membranous esophagitis, severe stenosis, infiltration of the esophageal wall, peptic ulcer distal to the stenosis (rarely visible)	Severe, irregular stenosis 5–10 cm above the diaphragm; hyperperistalsis with funnel-shaped deformity of the stomach below the stenosis, therefore no, or only small, hiatus hernia; immediately below the stenosis, a penetrating ulcer or "diverticulum" (not always visible)	Extended ulceration of the lower esophagus with stenosis by severe submucosal weal in and above the stenosis; scarring periesophagitis; penetrating callous ulcer at the junction of gastric and esophageal epithelium
IV	Same as stage III, but severe complications by progression as perforation of the ulcer into the mediastinum, pleura, or cardiac atrium or ventricle or malignant degeneration (adenosarcoma)		

(Wienbeck et al. 1976). In some cases purely conservative treatment is sufficient (Carre 1954; Prinsen 1975); in others the peptic stenosis is treated by fundoplication and dilatation and possibly a myotomy, as well. Extreme cases could require a resection with colonic interposition.

In recent decades since Barrett's publication (Barrett 1951) and apart from superficial biopsies of the mucous membrane (Paull et al. 1976, cited Postlethwaith and Sealy 1978), only a few reports on histological changes can be found on the resected esophagus in peptic stenoses in children. Therefore, some cases should be demonstrated, where the attempted fundoplication with myotomy and mobilization failed and a resection had to be carried out.

Case Reports

There were three patients between 14 months and 4 years of age in whom organ-conserving operative therapy had not brought about an improvement, as shown in Table 3. For this reason, a resection with colonic interposition had to be performed.

Case 1. Z.F., a 4-year-old boy; roentgenogram showed a short esophagus, (stage III) with a clear niche formation of a penetrating ulcer inside the stenosis. The operation showed (Fig. 1a–e) a subaortic stenosis in the area of the inflammed esophagus with severe periesophagitis, so that this area had to be resected. This region showed macroscopically extensive ulcerous esophagitis with flat ulcerations, a submucousal weal in the same area above the stenosis, just below it a

Table 3. Therapy of patients with resected Barrett's ulcer in childhood

Name and age at onset of therapy	Duration of dysphagia	Therapy			
Z.F., 4 years (Fig. 1a–c)	3 years (asthma)	Fundoplication + bougienage (Fig. 1a)	→ Additional gastrostomy 3 mon	→ Progress of stenosis, and Barrett's ulcer (Fig. 1b)	→ Resection + colonic interposition
A.E., 4 years (Fig. 2a)	6 weeks	Gastrostomy 3 mon	→ Progress of stenosis	→ Resection + colonic interposition	
M.S., 8 mon (Fig. 2b)	3 mon	Gastrostomy + fundoplication + bougienage 3 mon	→ Progress of stenosis Transthoracic "myotomy" + fundoplication due to perforation	→ Dehiscence Empyema Resection Esophagostoma	→ Colonic interposition

penetrating peptic ulcer, and adjacent to it macroscopically *normal* gastric mucous membrane (Fig. 1a, e).

The corresponding histological specimen cut longitudinally showed extensive damage of the submucosa which reached the esophageal muscle layer, with squamous epithelium in this area. Below the penetrating ulceration, normal *gastric mucosa of the fundus type, with parietal and chief cells,* was entirely intrathoracically situated (Fig. 1e).

Case 2. A.E., a 4-year-old boy; roentgenogram (Fig. 2a) showed no improvement after a gastrostomy. An ulcer-niche was evident under the area of stenosis, similar to case No. 1. Resection and colonic interposition were carried out. The resected lower esophagus in the thoracic area showed, on histological examination, an extended weal destroying the muscularis propria of the esophagus. Below the stenosis was *normal gastric mucous membrane with normally formed fundus glands and abundant chief, parietal and adjacent cells.*

Case 3. M.S., a 14-month-old girl; roentgenogram (Fig. 2b) showed a short esophagus (stage II–III). There was no improvement after gastrostomy; during an attempted myotomy the stenosis was perforated. It was covered by means of a fundoplication. Later, on a disruption required resection of the esophagus and colonic interposition.

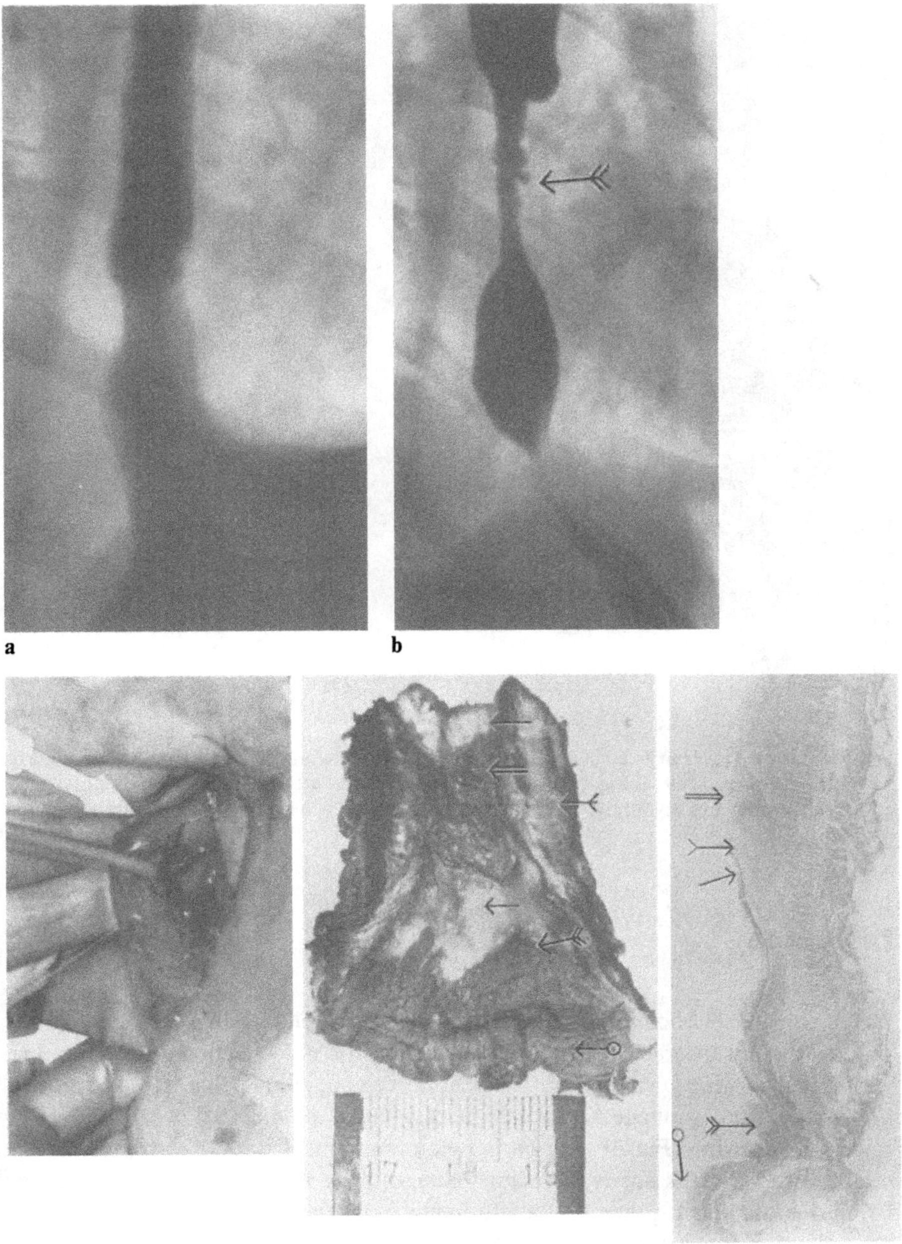

Fig. 1a–e. Barrett's ulcer in childhood, in Z.F., a 4-year-old boy. **a** 11.1.67: Improvement after gastrostomy. **b** 11.4.67: Ascending stenosis with penetrating ulcer (↗). **c** Situs during surgery: stenosis diaphragma. Resected area between *arrows*. **d** Resected specimen of esophagus. **e** Histologic specimen; ↗ squamous epithelium; ⇗ flat ulcerations; ↗ submucosal weal and destruction of muscularis; ♂ gastric epithelium; ↗ penetrating ulcer (Barrett's ulcer)

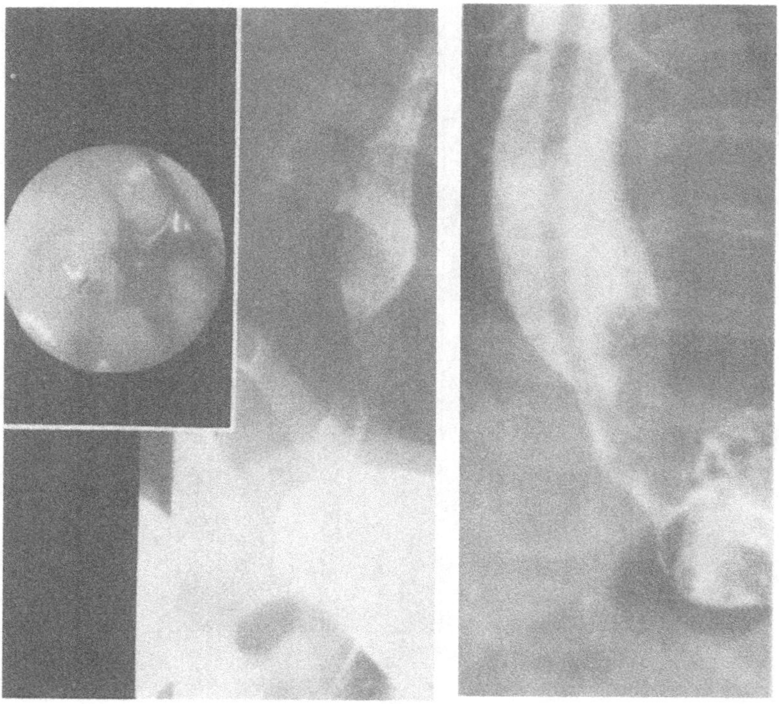

a b

Fig. 2. a Barrett's ulcer in A.E., a 4-year-old boy. No improvement after gastrostomy, leading to a penetrating ulcer (same as Fig. 1). **b** Barrett's ulcer in M.S., a 14-mo-old girl. No improvement after gastrostomy and myotomy. Eventual perforation of a penetrating ulcer during attempted myotomy

Discussion

In the original publication of Barrett (1951) the esophagus of a 13-year-old boy showed the intrathoracically situated normal gastric mucous membrane (Fig. 3a), with a perforating ulcer in the substenotic region; above this, flat ulcerations destroying the esophageal mucosa; and a clear submucosal weal, shown in schematic drawing (Fig. 3b). In earlier examinations of resected specimens from adults with Barrett's ulcers, the same changes were found, mainly characterized by flat, often fibrin-covered, longitudinally positioned ulcers in the squamous epithelium of the esophagus, with severe inflammation of the esophageal wall. In later stages there were extended, often circular, but always flat ulcerations in the lowest part of the esophagus, which ended caudally in tonguelike formations with bleeding and pseudomembranous fibrin coatings (Fig. 3c).

There were stenoses in this area, with heavy submucosal weals, mainly developed cranially to the stenosis (ascending fibrosis, according to K. Brown) (Kelly

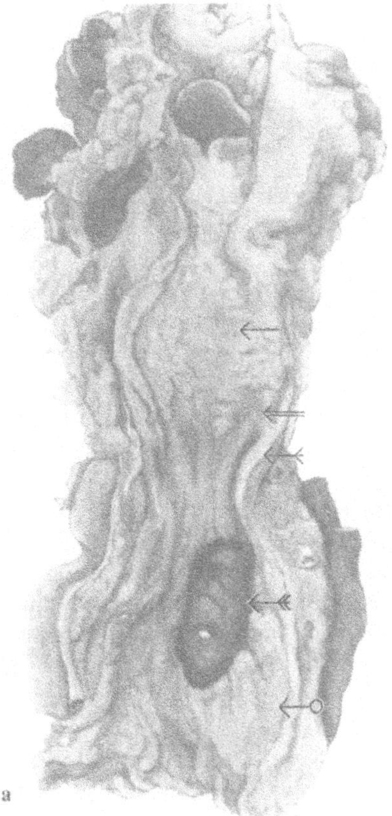

a

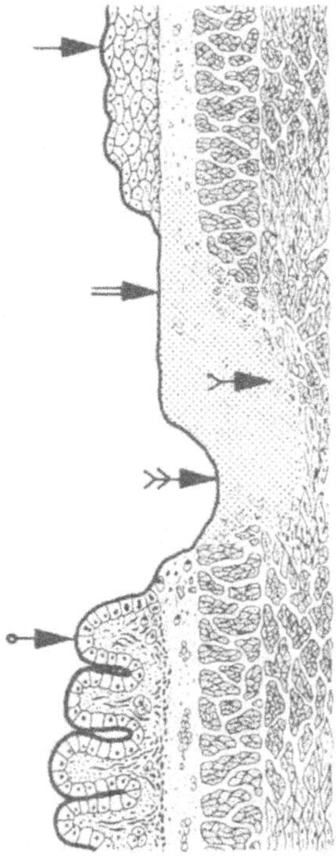

b

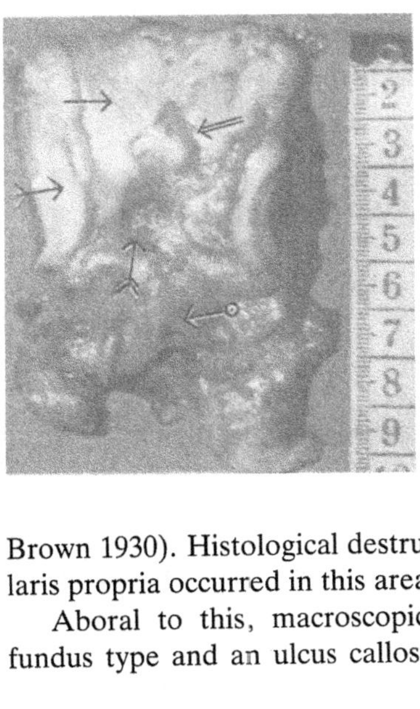

c

Fig. 3a. Original specimen from Barrett's first publication (1951). **b** Scheme of morphological structures and destructions. **c** Specimen from an adult with Barrett's ulcer. ↗ Squamous epithelium of the esophagus; ↗ superficial ulceration in the "lower esophagus"; ↗ weal of the submucosa and destruction of the muscularis propria; ↗ penetrating Barrett's ulcer (marginal ulceration) (Wolf et al. 1953, 1958); ♂ gastric mucosa (intrathoracic)

Brown 1930). Histological destruction and scarring of the submucosa and muscularis propria occurred in this area (Figs. 1a–e, 3b).

Aboral to this, macroscopically gastric mucous membrane of cardia and fundus type and an ulcus callosum penetrans of the peptic ulcer type could be found on the gastroesophageal epithelium (Barrett's ulcer, marginal ulceration, according to Wolf, Marshall, and Som) (Barrett 1951; Huber 1959; Kelly Brown 1930; Moersch 1948; Wolf et al. 1955, 1958; Wurnig 1955a, 1971) (Figs. 1d, c, 3b, c). These changes are regularly found in adults and can also be seen in resection specimens of children. This was also described by Kelly and Forshall (Kelly Brown 1930; Forshall 1955).

The progression of these changes was first described in children by Kelly Brown (1930) as a so-called *ascending esophageal fibrosis*. This was also obvious in our first case (Fig. 1a, b).

The best name, which recognizes the special localization of the callous ulceration, is that of Wolf, Marshall and Som (Wolf et al. 1955, 1958) (peptic esophageal stenosis with marginal ulceration; Table 1), whereby the submucosal stenosing scar is the "peptic esophageal stenosis" and the "marginal ulceration" denotes the constant penetrating peptic ulcer on the esophageal-gastric mucous membrane border, while the flat ulcerations in the upper esophagus are not specially mentioned.

To evaluate the condition endoscopically, the staging of Savary (Savary and Miller 1976) can be referred to. It must be mentioned, however, that according to the original presentation by Barrett, the actual Barrett's ulcer (marginal ulcer) may not be completely seen, or may not be seen at all, because it is below the stenosis (Figs. 1b–e, 3a–c). Only the flat ulcerations within the area of squamous epithelium above and in the stenosis may be visible (Fig. 3a, c).

The comparison of our resection specimens with those from adults shows identical relations, which are schematically shown in Fig. 3b, c. The progressive process can be divided into four stages, whereby the first three stages of the short esophagus are equivalent to Savary's four stages of reflux esophagitis (Savary and Miller 1976) (Table 2).

Evaluation in the Light of Operative Procedure

Besides the demonstrated progress without therapy (K. Brown, Forshall, our own patients), there are also patients that recover considerably, even after gastrostomy alone (Wurnig 1955a) and Hofmann (personal communication), and one of our own patients with leukemia. On the other hand the endoscopic stage IV according to Savary (Savary and Miller 1976) (our stage III) does not heal, and above all the development into stage IV with its terminal complications must be avoided (Table 2).

The morphological changes in advanced cases (stage III) are largely uniform, so that myotomy for elimination of the stenosis could easily, if not certainly, lead to the perforation of the esophagus (case 3). In contrast to cardiac achalasia, where the stenosis is situated in the muscular region, the peptic stenosis is situated in the submucosa; in addition in this area flat ulcerations of the esophageal mucous membrane can occur, so that after the splitting of the submucosal scar which forms the stenosis, the esophageal lumen is already perforated.

The dilatation of the peptic stenosis alone is not sufficient if the development has gone so far that in the substenotic area *gastric mucous membrane with parietal and chief cells* can be found. In these cases a progression, in spite of dilatation and fundoplication, can be expected, as we see in our patient, Z.F., case 1.

When one is evaluating these patients, a penetrating ulcer in the stenosis or below must be searched for carefully. If an ulcer can be found, the organ-preserving, semiconservative procedure is of no use.

We mentioned the disposition to carcinoma of a endobrachyesophagus with Barrett's ulcer as early as 1963 (Wurnig 1963). In the meantime this has been confirmed and is of special consideration in childhood (Smithers 1950; Wienbeck et al. 1976). Thus a careful follow-up examination is necessary in these cases.

To conclude this section on indications for operation and the type of operation, it must be emphasized that it is most important to apply the therapy as effectively as possible and as soon as possible, before an irreversible stage is reached. Certainly at stage I and probably at stage II, conservative measures can be carried out if they are done intensively and exactly enough. At stage II, organ-preserving surgical measures are certainly sufficient. In a definite stage III (endobrachyesophagus with Barrett's ulcer, peptic esophageal stenosis with marginal ulceration, only colonic interposition can be carried out in children as a long-term solution, if the morphological findings of resected specimens are taken into consideration. The attempt to cure the disease with organ-preserving operations, such as dilatation of the stenosis and fundoplication or similar procedures, would require at least careful long-term check-ups because of the danger of a progression to stage IV, according to our scheme.

Summary

The morphological findings in three resected specimens of Barrett's ulcer in children are discussed. Nearly identical morphologic changes are found in all cases, even in adults. This pathologic condition is understood as the third or fourth stage of reflux esophagitis. Perforation or even malignant degeneration is described in these cases. Therefore mainly all therapeutic aims must be to prevent these stages.

Résumé

Les auteurs décrivent les modifications morphologiques de l'œsophage chez l'enfant à partir de trois observations de résection œsophagienne pour ulcère de Barrett (endo-brachyœsophage avec ulcère de Barrett).

Ces lésions sont identiques tous les cas et parfaitement comparables aux lésions correspondantes chez l'adulte. Ces lésions sont à considérer comme stade III ou IV de l'œsophagite par reflux du fait que les stades I–III d'œsophage court correspondent aux stades I–IV d'œsophagite par reflux d'après Savary. Les auteurs insistent sur la difficulté de diagnostiquer l'ulcère de Barrett lui-même car il est dans presque tous les cas situé en dessous de la sténose et de ce fait non visible ou très difficilement visible par endoscopie. Le rôle des mesures thérapeutiques dans ce domaine est d'éviter l'évolution des stades III en stade IV avec perforation de l'ulcère ou dégénerescence maligne.

Zusammenfassung

Anhand von 3 Fällen resezierter Barrett-Ulzera des Ösophagus im Kindesalter (Endobrachyösophagus mit Barrett-Ulkus) werden die morphologischen Veränderungen beschrieben. Sie sind in allen Fällen nahezu identisch, auch im Vergleich mit den entsprechenden Veränderungen beim Erwachsenen.

Der Zustand wird als Stadium III oder Stadium IV der Refluxösophagitis aufgefaßt, wobei die Stadien I–III des kurzen Ösophagus den Stadien I–IV der Refluxösophagitis nach Savary entsprechen. Auf die Schwierigkeit, das Barrett-Ulkus selbst zu diagnostizieren, wird hingewiesen, da es typischerweise in nahezu allen Fällen unterhalb der Stenose gelegen und daher endoskopisch nur sehr schwer oder gar nicht einsehbar ist. Da in diesen Fällen des Stadiums III des kurzen Ösophagus, die Weiterentwicklung ins Stadium IV mit Perforation des Ulkus oder maligner Degeneration möglich ist und mehrfach beobachtet wurde, ist das therapeutische Rüstzeug darauf auszurichten, die Entwicklung dieser Stadien zu verhindern.

References

Adlersberg D, Som M (1956) Esophagitis and esophageal ulcer. Med Clin North Am 40

Allison PR (1948) Peptic ulcer of the oesophagus. Thorax 3:20

Allison PR (1949) Oesophagus. Br Surg Pract 6:315–353

Allison PR, Johnstone AS (1953) The oesophagus lined with gastric mucous membrane. Thorax 8:87

Barrett NR (1951) Chronic peptic ulcer of the oesophagus and "oesophagitis". Br J Surg 38:175

Boix-Ochoa I, Rehbein F (1965) Oesophageal stenosis due to reflux oesophagitis. Arch Dis Child 40:197

Carre AR (1954) Gastroesophageal incompetence in children. Radiology 62:351

Forshall I (1955) The cardio-oesophageal syndrome in childhood. Arch Dis Child 30:46

Franklin RH, Henderson ID (1955) Two cases of oesophageal stricture in childhood requiring resection. Arch Dis Child 30:55

Huber P (1959) Angeborene Oesophagusstenose oder Narbenstenose nach Refluxoesophagitis? Wien Klin Wochenschr 71:950

Kelly A Brown (1930) Congenital stenosis of the esophagus in children associated with diaphragmatic hernia of the stomach. J Laryngol Otol 45:680

Konrad RM, Rotthof F (1959) Der Brachyesophagus (Pathogenese, Diagnose und Klinik des angeborenen und erworbenen kurzen Oesophagus). Bruns Beitr Klin Chir 198:448

Moersch HJ (1948) Diskussionsbemerkungen zu Benedikt EB und Sweet RH: Benign stricture of the oesophagus. Gastroenterology 11:627

Monereo J, Corte L, Blasa E (1975) Peptic esophageal stenosis in children. J Pediatr Surg 8:478

Paull A, Trier SJ, Dalton D, et al (1976) The histologic spectrum of Barrett's esophagus. N Engl J Med 295:476

Postlethwaith RW, Sealy WC (1978) Surgery of the esophagus. Appleton-Century Crofts, New York, p 40

Prinsen JE (1975) Hiatus hernia in infants and children: a long-term follow-up of medical treatment. J Pediatr Surg 10:97

Savary M, Miller G (1976) Endoskopische Befunde bei der Ösophagitis. In: Siewert R, Blum AL, Waldeck F (Hrsg) Funktionsstörungen der Speiseröhre. Springer, Berlin Heidelberg New York, S 223–253

Shmerling DH (1976) Funktionsstörungen der Speiseröhre im Kindesalter. In: Siewert R, Blum AL, Waldeck F (Hrsg) Funktionsstörungen der Speiseröhre. Springer, Berlin Heidelberg New York

Smithers DW (1950) The association of cancer of the gastric cardia with partial thoracic stomach, short esophagus and peptic ulceration. J Radiol 23:261

Wienbeck M, Heitmann P, Sievert R, Rossetti M (1976) Endobrachyoesophagus und peptische Oesophagusstenosen. In: Siewert R, Blum AL, Waldeck F (Hrsg) Funktionsstörungen der Speiseröhre. Springer, Berlin Heidelberg New York

Wolf BS, Marshall RH, Som ML (1953) Short esophagus with esophagogastric or marginal ulceration. Radiology 61:473

Wolf BS, Marshall RH, Som ML, Winkelstein A (1955) Peptic esophagitis and peptic ulcer of the esophagus and marginal esophagogastric ulceration. Gastroenterology 29:744

Wolf BS, Marshall RH, Som ML (1958) Peptic esophagitis and peptic ulceration of the esophagus. Am J Roentgenol 79:741

Wurnig P (1955a) Die intrathoracale Verlagerung der Cardia ohne Hiatushernie. Thoraxchirurgie 3:111

Wurnig P (1955b) Über krebsdisponierende Zustände an Ösophagus und Cardia. Dtsch Z Chir 280:504

Wurnig P (1963) Der kurze Ösophagus. Thoraxchir Cardiovasc Chir 10:527

Wurnig P (1971) Die Eigenheiten der Hiatushernie im Kindesalter, Formen, Indikation und Art der Operation. Pädiatr Pädol 6:188

Combined Disturbance of Respiratory Regulation and Esophageal Function in Early Infancy*

R. Kurz[1], M. Höllwarth[1], M. Fasching[1], R. Haidmayer[2], K. P. Pfeiffer[2], and T. Kenner[2]

Introduction

Studies of central respiratory regulation disturbances (Haidmayer et al. 1982b) and esophageal motor functioning (Höllwarth 1979) in infants, which have been done independently of one another, called our attention to the frequent coincidence of apnea during sleep and gastroesophageal reflux (GER). Since both frequent and long periods of sleep apnea (Guilleminault and Ariagno 1977; Haidmayer et al. 1982a, b; Naeye 1977; Southall et al. 1980; Steinschneider 1972) as well as gastroesophageal reflux (Downing and Lee (1975; Herbst et al. 1978, 1979; Lawson 1981; Leape et al. 1977; Ramenofsky and Leape 1981) are associated with the sudden death syndrome (SIDS), we tried to establish the coincidence of both disorders quantitatively.

Methods

In 43 infants between the ages of 1 and 18 weeks, we performed impedance pneumography and esophageal manometry. The impedance pneumography was accomplished using a strip chart recorder (Hellige) throughout at least 1 hour of sleep. The length and frequency of the apneic episodes were read from the recording curve and stored in a digital computer (Hewlett Packard 2100A). The length of the interruptions in breathing during sleep are expressed by the mean apnea length (MA) values.

$$\text{MA (s/min)} = \frac{\text{total apnea duration (s)}}{\text{period of recording (min)}} \text{ (Haidmayer et al. 1982a, b).}$$

Infants, whose breathing during sleep repeatedly stopped for no clear reason and resulted in cyanosis of various intensities, were classified as risk cases with clinically evident apneas during sleep. Some of them needed artificial respiratory help (the so-called near miss infants). Like in earlier reports, apneas in risk cases appeared more frequently and mostly periodically with the maximum duration of the single apneic phases being generally longer than 10 s.

The esophageal manometry was done on unprepared patients as a three-point pressure measurement with continous perfusion (0.2–0.5 ml 5% glucose) using a

* Supported by Grant No. 2883 from the "Fonds zur Förderung der wissenschaftlichen Forschung in Österreich".

1 Univ.-Klinik für Kinderchirurgie, Heinrichstraße 31, A-8010 Graz/Austria
2 Physiologisches Institut der Karl-Franzens-Universität, Harrachgasse 21, A-8010 Graz/Austria

Progress in Pediatric Surgery, Vol. 18
Ed. by P. Wurnig

Table 1. Age and weight data for the three groups of patients

	Age (weeks)	Weight (g)	Birth weight (g)	Gestational age (weeks)
Group A	5	3570	2980	36.5
($n=10$)	(1–14)	(2830–4500)	(1800–4300)	(28–39.5)
Group B	7	4060	3071	37.0
($n=12$)	(1–14)	(2090–7680)	(1040–3950)	(28–40)
Group C	6	3373	2671	35
($n=21$)	(1–18)	(2170–5720)	(850–4950)	(27–40)

Group A, control group
Group B, infants with recurrent vomiting
Group C, infants with prolonged sleep apneas

high-pressure perfusion pump. First, several pressure profiles of the lower esophageal sphincter (LES) were taken. Following that, two measuring points were placed in the esophagus and a third in the stomach. The spontaneous esophageal motor function as well as the common cavity phenomenon as a manographic reflux manifestation were registered. We considered more than three common cavity phases of more than 10 s or one phase of more than 15 s to be a pathological reflux. Finally, all three measuring points were placed in the esophagus, and the esophageal motor function was evaluated according to the mean number of regular and propulsive peristaltic waves that occurred following ten swallows. Fewer than seven propulsive swallowing waves after ten swallows was considered to be a sign of disturbed esophageal motor function.

The 43 infants were divided into three groups and compared to one another (Table 1). Ten infants made up the healthy control group A, and 12 infants with the clinical symptom "recurrent spitting up" or "vomiting" were in group B. Later, clinically manifest sleep apnea appeared in one of these infants. In the third group, there were 22 infants who came to our attention primarily because of clinically manifest, prolonged sleep apnea. After examining their histories, seven of these infants were found to have recurrent vomiting.

In all of the infants, information, such as duration of pregnancy, birth weight, weight and age at the time of testing, and the history of perinatal complications (asphyxia, idiopathic respiratory distress syndrome (IRDS), and adaptation disturbances), was noted. The statistical calculations were done using Student's *t* test.

Results

The three groups were comparable with regard to birth weight, length of gestation, and age and weight at the time of testing (Table 1). In the control infant group (group A), the mean MA value of 3.2 ± 1.3 s/min was in the normal range,

Table 2. MA values, cardial pressure, gastroesophageal reflux, and peristalsis

	MA values (s/min)			Cardial pressure (mmHg)	Gastro-esophageal reflux (n)	Peristalsis	
A ($n=10$)	3.2 ± 1.3			21.6 ± 11.6	1	9.2 ± 1.6	
		N.S.					
B ($n=12$)	5.5 ± 4.4		H.S.	23.8 ± 10.4	8	8.4 ± 1.7	L.S.
		S.					
C ($n=21$)	13.3 ± 7.9			22.3 ± 7.0	14	7.5 ± 1.4	

N.S., no significance
S., significant ($P<0.01$)
H.S., high significance ($P<0.001$)
L.S., low significance ($P<0.05$)

Table 3. Gestational age versus MA values, gastroesophageal reflux, and esophageal peristalsis

Gestational age		MA value (s/min)		Gastro-esophageal reflux (n)	Peristalsis	
≤ 36 weeks	With control group	12.2 ± 8.6		12	7.7 ± 1.7	
($n=21$)	Without control group	14.2 ± 8.5		12	7.0 ± 1.3	
			S.			L.S.
			S.			
> 36 weeks	With control group	5.8 ± 4.3		11	8.4 ± 1.6	
($n=22$)	Without control group	6.9 ± 4.4		10	8.4 ± 1.5	

S., significant ($P<0.01$)
L.S., low significance ($P<0.05$)

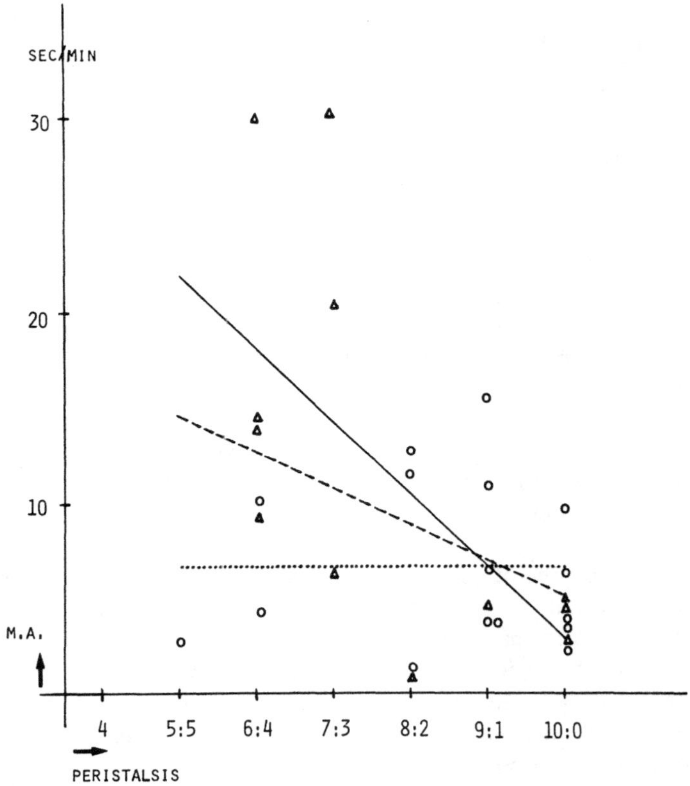

Fig. 1. Correlation between MA values and esophageal peristalsis in infants of less than/or 36-weeks gestation (———, △; $n=12$), in infants of more than 36-weeks gestation (·······, ○; $n=18$), and in all infants (-----; $n=30$)

as compared with 230 control infants of the same age who were tested in an earlier study (MA = 2.97 ± 2.13 s/min). The cardial pressure values were normal. Peristalsis showed no pathological contractions. A pathological reflux (GER) was apparent in one patient (Table 2).

In the group with recurrent spitting up (group B), the mean MA value of 5.5 ± 4.4 s/min was higher than in group A, but still significantly lower ($P<0.01$) than in group C. The cardial pressure values remained normal, irrespective of the length of gestation, birth weight, and age at the time of testing. Propulsive peristalsis was, on the average, worse than in group A, but a significant difference could not be proved. Eight of the 12 patients showed a pathological reflux, and in four, the reflux phases appeared particularly often (Table 2).

Group C (with clinically manifest sleep apnea) had a high mean MA value (13.3 ± 7.9 s/min), which was significantly higher than that of group B ($P<0.01$) and that of group A ($P<0.001$). The cardial pressure values were normal. Peristalsis was slightly poorer than in the control group ($P<0.05$). However, patho-

Table 4. Perinatal complications versus incidence of prolonged sleep apneas and gastroesophageal reflux

Perinatal complications	Prolonged sleep apneas	Gastroesophageal reflux
With ($n=16$)	10 (62.5%)	9 (56.3%)
Without ($n=27$)	12 (44.4%)	14 (51.9%)

logical contractions occurred definitely more often. Pathological reflux episodes were apparent in two-thirds of the patients in groups B and C (Table 2).

When considering all the groups, and using the length of gestation as the point of reference, significantly higher MA values ($P<0.01$) were found in premature babies (gestation less than 36 weeks) than in full-term newborns (Table 3). The esophageal motor function was slightly poorer ($P<0.05$) in newborns. The occurrence of reflux was, however, not related to the length of gestation. Also with regard to birth weight and weight and age at the time of testing, the reflux showed no preference.

The comparison of the degree of pathological peristalsis and the length of the MA values showed no correlation for full-term infants (Fig. 1). In addition, the statistical comparison between pathological reflux episodes and MA values showed a positive correlation only for premature babies. The checking of the time relationship between apnea and reflux revealed that sporadic apnea occurs more often in connection with reflux, while periodical apnea could more often be observed independently of reflux episodes.

In infants with perinatal complications, clinically evident sleep apnea occurred in 62.5%, and in 44.4% of children without perinatal complications. Infants with and without reflux showed no difference of this kind (Table 4).

Discussion

Numerous studies point out that the so-called sudden infant death syndrome is caused in most cases by defective respiratory regulation which manifest itself in increased and extended apnea during sleep (Brady et al. 1978; Guilleminault and Ariagno 1977; Haidmayer et al. 1982a, b; Naeye 1977; Rigatto 1977b; Steinschneider 1972). Recent studies reveal that sleep apnea and gastroesophageal reflux (GER) are closely related. Leape et al. (1977), Herbst et al. (1978, 1979), and Ramenofsky and Leape (1981) detected a gastroesophageal reflux in near miss infants revived at the last minute. This was also the case in two-thirds of our infants with clinically evident sleep apneas.

Every high-rising gastroesophageal reflux is capable of causing reflex pauses in breathing (Lawson 1981). Sutton et al. (1978) showed, in research on animals, that irreversible central apnea can be caused by electrical stimulation of the

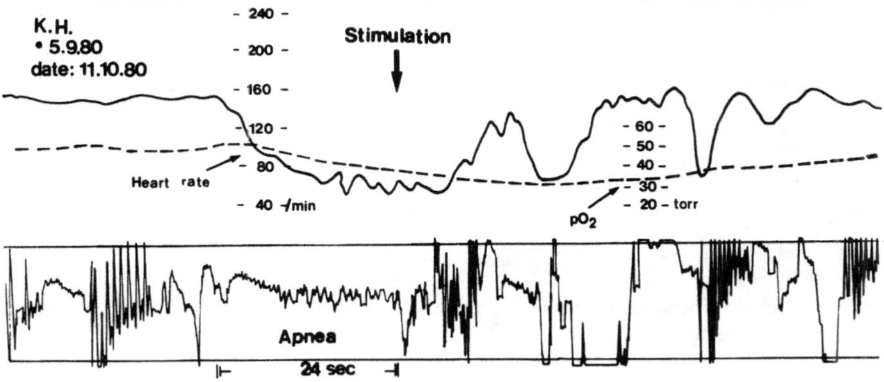

Fig. 2. Fortuitous recording of a near miss event

superior laryngeal nerve, depending on the stimulation intensity. Herbst et al. (1978) achieved a similar effect in infants by putting acidic fluid in the upper esophagus. Downing and Lee (1975) and Lee et al. (1977) caused apnea in piglets with water and cow's milk. Harned et al. (1978) demonstrated similar results in lambs. This, however, was not reproducible in infants (Herbst et al. 1979). Pinkham and Beckwith (1970) found vocal cord lesions in infants who died of SIDS, which, however, were not described by other authors (i.e., Althoff 1980). Like Herbst (1979), we found that only some of the children with gastroesophageal reflux also showed clinical symptoms of "recurrent vomiting."

Based on the presented results, the relationship between apnea and gastroesophageal reflux can be defined as follows: the tendency to develop apnea as a result of a defective respiratory regulation during sleep and disturbed esophageal motor function are related to the degree of maturity of the patient. Therefore, both symptoms are evidence of a regulatory immaturity. Although the incidence of reflux in this study does not run parallel to immaturity, the frequency of reflux rises with the increase in disturbed esophageal paristalsis. The increased incidence of reflux and disturbed esophageal motor function in children with clinically evident sleep apnea indicates that in some infants, a combined regulatory immaturity of the autonomic centers persists.

The explanation for the fact that the clinical manifestation of sleep apnea is fostered by gastroesophageal reflux is found in the characteristics of respiratory regulation in these infants. After apnea caused by reflux, the pO_2 in the blood decreases slightly temporarily. The risk that the rise of the pO_2 will be delayed, or that repeated apeneic episodes will go into a threatening respiratory arrest, is greater the more pronounced the tendency to spontaneous apnea. By means of respiratory answer curves, we found that low-grade hypoxia during sleep in some of the infants led not to the expected stimulation but to a paradoxical respiratory depression and provoked periodical apnea which was not primarily connected to reflux (Haidmayer et al. 1982a). This paradoxical breathening behavior (detected in newborns by Rigatto (1977a, b) is more distinct in risk infants with sleep apnea

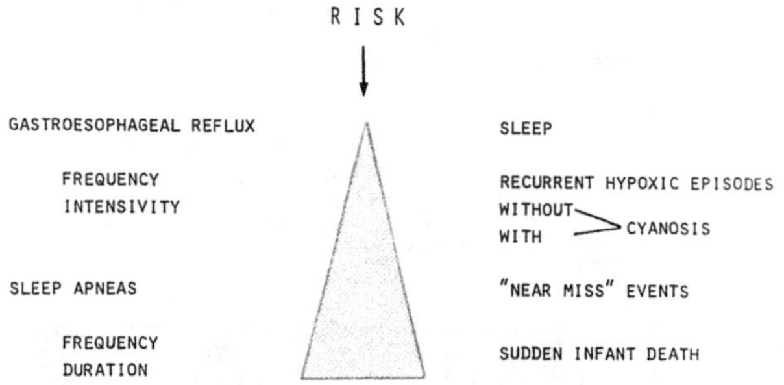

Fig. 3. Risk relations between esophageal function and central respiratory regulation with regard to sudden infant death

syndrome (Haidmayer et al. 1982a). Brady et al. (1978) found a similar effect of hypoxemia in near miss infants. By accident, we were able to register a near miss event in an infant in whom the tendency to apnea and the frequency of reflux were especially pronounced (Fig. 2). Together with visible but low-grade vomiting, there was a spontaneous, irreversible respiratory arrest with increasing bradycardia and a gradual decrease of the transcutaneously registered pO_2. Only by respiratory stimulation, was this condition able to be corrected.

Based on these results, it follows that the risk of a reflex apnea accompanied by gastroesophageal reflux increases in proportion to the disturbance in the central respiratory regulation present at the same time, whereby frequency and intensity of the reflux are also influential (Fig. 3) and can play a dangerous role by themselves in some cases (Ariagno and Guilleminault 1982). The stability of the respiratory regulation is related to the immaturity of the child and to the perinatal complications and manifests itself mostly within the first months of life during sleeping. Sleep itself creates a slight suppression in breathing, whereby the breath-stimulating sensory impulses which are transmitted by the reticular formation while awake are not active. Still it must be supposed that gastroesophageal reflux presents only one of various possible factors causing respiratory depression and hypoxia. The same effect in an obstruction of the nasal passages (Stark and Thach 1976), e.g., in inflammations of the upper airways, toxic-septic conditions, or postanesthesia sleep (Kurz et al. 1983), combined with the basic defect in a disturbed respiratory regulation, must be considered as a realization factor of SIDS.

The possibility for an effective prophylaxis consists in treating the apneic tendency with aminophylline, in analogy to the treatment of apneas in preterm newborns (Gabriel et al. 1978; Myers et al. 1980), and the treatment of reflux by elevating the upper body and thickening the nourishment given. The 14 near miss infants described by Herbst (1979) had no more respiratory disturbances after they were placed in an elevated position. On the other hand, one patient died of SIDS after the parents arbitrarily discontinued treatment of the reflux. Ramenofsky (1981) found that in two-thirds of the patients, a lying-on-the-stomach position had a better effect than the usual sitting position at 60° in the hiatus chair. One of our own known risk cases died suddenly in the night. In this case, a partial paralysis of the diaphragm was an additional risk factor. In the remaining patients, the respiratory type normalized by the 6th month of life and the reflux function within the 1st year.

Summary

An evident coincidence exists between increased and extended apneas during sleep and frequent gastroesophageal reflux as well as disturbances of propulsive esophageal peristalsis. The tendency to develop apnea and disturbed esophageal function are related to the degree of the maturity of the patient. This indicates that in some infants, a combined regulatory immaturity of the autonomic centers persists. Moreover, the gastroesophageal reflux fosters the clinical manifestation of sleep apneas. The risk of a reflex apnea accompanied by gastroesophageal reflux increases in proportion to the disturbance in the central respiratory regulation present at the same time. This pathomechanism can be considered one of the causes of the sudden infant death syndrome.

The possibility of effective prophylaxis consists in treating the apneic tendency with aminophylline and the treatment of reflux by elevating the upper body and thickening the nourishment given.

Résumé

Il existe une coincidence significative entre apnées de sommeil fréquentes et prolongées, reflux gastro-œsophagien et troubles du mouvement péristaltique. La tendance à l'apnée et aux troubles fonctionnels de l'œsophage dépend du degré de maturité du patient. Cela semble indiquer que chez certains nourrissons, il persiste une immaturité des centres autonomes de régulation. En outre, le reflux gastro-œsophagien peut faciliter l'apparition du symptôme clinique de l'apnée de sommeil.

Le risque qu'un reflux gastro-œsophagien entraine une apnée de sommeil réflexe est d'autant plus grand que les troubles éventuellement pré-existants de la régulation respiratoire centrale sont plus sérieux. Ce mécanisme pathologique peut être considéré comme une des causes de la mort subite des nourrissons.

Pour une prophylaxie efficace, on traitera la tendance á l'apnée à l'aminophylline, on mettra l'enfant en position assise et on épaissira les aliments.

Zusammenfassung

Es besteht eine auffällige Koinzidenz von gehäuften und verlängerten Schlafapnoen und vermehrtem gastroösophagealem Reflux sowie einer Störung der propulsiven Ösophagusmotorik. Apnoeneigung und gestörte Ösophagusfunktion stehen in Beziehung zum Reifegrad der Patienten. Dies spricht dafür, daß bei einigen Säuglingen eine kombinierte Regulationsunreife autonomer Zentren persistiert.

Darüber hinaus vermag ein gastroösophagealer Reflux die klinische Manifestation von Schlafapnoen zu begünstigen. Das Risiko einer den gastroösophagealen Reflux begleitenden reflektorischen Apnoe steigt mit dem Grad der gleichzeitig vorliegenden zentralen Atemregulationsstörung an. Dieser Pathomechanismus kann als eine der Ursachen des plötzlichen Kindestodes angesehen werden. Die Möglichkeit einer Prophylaxe besteht in der Behandlung der Apnoeneigung mit Aminophyllin und der Refluxbehandlung mit Hochlagerung des Kindes und Eindicken der Nahrung.

References

Althoff H (1980) Sudden infant death syndrome (SIDS). Forensic-medical experience, research and conclusions regarding a general medical problem. Fischer, Stuttgart

Ariagno RL, Guilleminault C (1982) Movement and gastroesophageal reflux in awake term infants with "near miss" SIDS, unrelated to apnea. J Pediatr 100:894–897

Brady JP, Ariagno RL, Watts JL, Goldmann SL, Dumpit FM (1978) Apnea, hypoxemia and aborted sudden infant death syndrome. Pediatrics 62:686–691

Downing SE, Lee JC (1975) Laryngeal chemosensitivity: a possible mechanism for sudden infant death. Pediatrics 55:640–649

Gabriel M, Witolla C, Albam M (1978) Sleep and aminophylline treatment of apnea in preterm infants. Eur J Pediatr 128:145–149

Guilleminault C, Ariagno R (1977) Sudden infant death syndrome. Bull Eur Physiopathol Respir 13:591–597

Haidmayer R, Kurz R, Kenner T, Wurm H, Pfeiffer KP (1982a) Physiological and clinical aspects of respiration control in infants with relation to the sudden infant death syndrome. Klin Wochenschr 60:9–18

Haidmayer R, Pfeiffer KP, Kenner T, Kurz R (1982b) Statistical evaluation of respiratory control in infants to assess possible risk for the sudden infant death syndrome (SIDS). Eur J Pediatr 138:145–150

Harned SH, Myracle J, Ferreiro J (1978) Respiratory suppression and swallowing from introduction of fluids into the laryngeal region of the lamb. Pediatr Res 12:1003–1009

Herbst JJ, Book LS, Bray PF (1978) Gastroesophageal reflux in the "near miss" sudden infant death syndrome. J Pediatr 92:73–75

Herbst JJ, Minton SD, Book LS (1979) Gastroesophageal reflux causing respiratory distress and apnea in newborn infants. J Pediatr 95:763–768

Höllwarth M (1979) Die Entwicklung der Speiseröhrenfunktion bei Neugeborenen — eine manometrische Studie. Z Kinderchir 27:201–215

Kurz R, Schneeweiß S, Haidmayer R, Kenner T, Pfeiffer KP (1983) Früherkennung zentraler Atemregulationsstörungen beim Säugling zur Vermeidung postoperativer Komplikationen. Klin Pädiatr 195:29–32

Lawson EE (1981) Prolonged central respiratory inhibition following reflux-induced apnea. J Appl Physiol 50:874–879

Leape LL, Holder TM, Franklin JD, Amoury RA, Asheraft KW (1977) Respiratory arrest in infants secondary to gastroesophageal reflux. Pediatrics 60:924–927

Lee JC, Stoll BJ, Downing SE (1977) Properties of the laryngeal chemoreflux in neonatal piglets. Am J Physiol 233(1):R30–R36

Myers T, Milsap RL, Krauss AN, Auld PAM, Reidenberg MM (1980) Low-dose theophylline therapy in idiopathic apnea of prematurity. J Pediatr 96:99–103
Naeye RL (1977) The sudden infant death syndrome. Arch Pathol Lab Med 101:165–167
Pinkham JR, Beckwith JB (1970) Vocal cord lesions in the sudden infant death syndrome. In: Bergmann AB, Beckwith JB, Ray CG (eds) Proceedings of the 2nd international conference on causes of sudden infant death in infants. University of Washington Press, Seattle
Ramenofsky ML, Leape LL (1981) Continuous upper esophageal pH monitoring in infants and children with gastroesophageal reflux, pneumonia, and apneic spells. J Pediatr Surg 16: 374–378
Rigatto H (1977a) Ventilatory response to hypoxia. Semin Perinatol 1:357–362
Rigatto H (1977b) Apnea and periodic breathing. Semin Perinatol 1:375–381
Southall DP, Richards J, Brown DJ, Johnston PGB, De Swiet M, Shinebourne EA (1980) 24-hour tape recordings of ECG and respiration in the newborn infant with findings related to sudden death and unexplained brain damage in infancy. Arch Dis Child 55:7–16
Stark AR, Thach BT (1976) Mechanisms of airway obstruction leading to apnea in newborn infants. J Pediatr 89:982–985
Steinschneider A (1972) Prolonged apnea and the sudden infant death syndrome: clinical and laboratory observations. Pediatrics 50:646–654
Sutton D, Taylor EM, Lindemann RC (1978) Prolonged apnea in infant monkeys resulting from stimulation of superior laryngeal nerve. Pediatrics 61:519–527

Esophageal Dysfunction and Bronchial Asthma

G. KJELLÉN[1]

The diagnostic examination of the esophagus is commonly done by otolaryngologists in Sweden in contrast to the custom in the United States, for instance. My intention is to look at the relationship between esophageal dysfunction and bronchial asthma in adults.

The Swiss physician Mermod was the first to describe the connection between pulmonary and esophageal disease in 1887 (Mermod 1887).

In his original paper, he described a young woman with achalasia of the esophagus who complained of severe cough. In 1946, Mendelson described an asthmalike condition in patients who had aspirated during general anesthesia.

Several investigators mention the connection between asthma and gastroesophageal reflux (GER). Urschel and Paulson showed in 1967 that out of 636 patients with hiatus hernia and gastroesophageal reflux, 16% had asthma. As only 3% of the adult population suffers from asthma, the asthmatics are overrepresented in this group of patients. Mays (1976) found that 64% of his adult patients with asthma had hiatus hernias and 46% had a gastroesophageal reflux.

In children with asthma, Friedland et al. (1973) found hiatus hernias in 48%, and in a control group without asthma, he found only 14% with hiatus hernias. Therefore, many investigators tried to find microaspirations in asthmatic patients, but till now this was not possible, even with methods as sophisticated as scintigraphy, i.e., radioactive isotope activity was not found in the pulmonary fields after instillation into the stomach (Ghaed and Stein 1979).

There are reports showing that symptoms of asthma improved after conservative or surgical treatment of GER. Fonkalsrud (1980) showed that after Nissen's fundoplication asthma vanished in 13 of 14 children.

My own investigation was done in 97 adult asthmatic patients in 1981 (Kjellén 1981). Their average age was 53 years.

They were all patients of a pulmonary clinic, but in the stage of outpatient care and in clinical remission.

They answered a questionnaire and had an examination of the esophagus (manometry and an acid perfusion test) (Table 1).

Dynamic and static spirometry was also done. With manometry, we tried to detect hiatus hernias and dyskinesia of the esophagus, i.e., irregular contractions. We also tried to find cases with lowered pressure of the lower esophageal sphincter (under 6 mmHg). An acid perfusion test was also performed (i.e., by perfusion of the lower esophagus with diluted hydrochloric acid, we tried to evoke symptoms of reflux in the patient).

[1]Department of Otolaryngology, University Hospital, S-581 85 Linköping, Sweden

Progress in Pediatric Surgery, Vol. 18
Ed. by P. Wurnig

Table 1. Examinations performed and information obtained

Esophagomanometry	Hiatus hernia? Dyskinetic (nonperistaltic) contractions? Hypotension of the lower esophageal sphincter (< 6 mmHg)
Acid perfusion test (Bernstein test)	Positive?

Findings

In the 97 patients we investigated, we found dyskinesia in 38%, hiatus hernias in 37%, lowered pressure in the lower esophageal sphincter in 27%, and a positive acid perfusion test in 24% (Table 2).

Esophageal dysfunction was present in 67%. Esophageal dysfunction was more common in exogenous (95%) than in endogenous asthma (58%). Simultaneously with this study, a screening of the population was performed. As control patients, 55-year-old people from Linköping were selected at random and the function of their esophagus was tested. In this control group, 34% showed a dysfunction of the esophagus (Table 2). All differences between the two groups were significant. The symptoms reported by the patients with asthma are listed in Table 3.

Asthmatic patients with disturbed esophageal function had significantly more often the feeling of a lump in the throat, acid regurgitation, or retrosternal burning. They also had a feeling of overloading after meals and retrosternal pain when lying down, which ceased if the head end of the bed was raised.

Asthmatic patients with disturbed esophageal function had more severe bronchial symptomatology than asthmatics with a sound esophagus. Wheezing and massive expectoration were seen in 48% of the "esophagus" patients, compared with 19% of asthmatics with a sound esophagus (Table 4).

Table 2. Comparison of asthmatic patients and randomly selected persons 55 years of age

	Asthmatic patients ($n = 97$)	Incidentally elected patients of 55 years of age ($n = 209$)	
Hiatus hernia	37%	14%	$P<0.001$
Dyskinetic contractions	38%	17%	$P<0.001$
Hypotension of the lower esophageal sphincter	27%	5%	$P<0.001$
Positive acid perfusion test	24%	6%	$P<0.001$
Dysfunction of the esophagus in all	67%	34%	$P<0.001$

Table 3. Esophageal symptoms in 97 asthmatic patients

	Normal esophageal function ($n = 32$)	Dysfunction of the esophagus ($n = 65$)	
Sensation of globus	6%	42%	$P<0.001$
Dysphagia	16%	31%	NS
Overloaded sensation after meal	16%	40%	$P<0.05$
Regurgitation (heartburn)	19%	43%	$P<0.05$
Retrosternal pain during effort, vanishing after rest	25%	48%	NS
Retrosternal pain during cold weather	22%	42%	NS
Retrosternal pain when lying flat	3%	26%	$P<0.01$

Table 4. Respiratory symptoms

	Wheezing and cough with expectoration	
Normal esophageal function ($n = 32$)	19%	$P<0.05$
Esophageal dysfunction ($n = 65$)	46%	

The results of pulmonary function tests did not differ in the two groups. There was no difference in the amount and kind of drugs which were used. To find out if antireflux treatment is able to influence asthma, one half of asthmatic patients with dysfunction of the esophagus were placed into a treatment group (group 1) and the other half into a control of group (group 2).

In group 1, the following measures were taken:

1. The head end of the bed was raised 10 cm (without an extra pillow)
2. A glass of lukewarm water was drunk after every meal
3. No meals were allowed later than 3 h before going to sleep
4. All movements which were apt to raise the intraabdominal pressure were to be avoided
5. Gaviscon was given to prevent reflux

Group 2 had no such regimen at all, and the antiasthma durgs remained unchanged in both.

After 2 months another examination was done. No difference in pulmonary function tests was seen. On the other hand, the consumption of antiasthma drugs diminished and the esophageal function improved in the therapy group, but not in the control group. Furthermore, the patients in the therapy group reported improvement of esophageal symptoms, and of the bronchial complaints (Table 5). As no conclusions can be drawn from this or other observations, in view of aspira-

Table 5. Results of therapy in asthmatics with esophageal dysfunction

	Group with intensified therapy ($n = 31$)	Control group ($n = 31$)	
Improvement of esophageal dysfunction symptoms	87%	11%	$P<0.001$
Improvement of bronchial symptoms			
Dyspnea	54%	11%	$P<0.01$
Wheezing	48%	16%	$P<0.05$
Cough	46%	4%	$P<0.001$
Expectoration	52%	4%	$P<0.001$

tion one must assume other mechanisms of interaction between esophageal dysfunction and asthma.

A vagal nerve reflex between esophagus and bronchi might be such a mechanism. Therefore, the "single breath nitrogen" test was performed, which is a very sensitive test to detect obstruction in the small bronchi. Examination was performed in 15 asthmatic patients with a positive acid perfusion test. They were examined first before and then after acid perfusion of the esophagus and finally after application of acid-neutralizing drugs. It was found that under acid perfusion, the inclination of the alveolar plateau increased, and it diminished under neutralization (Fig. 1). This hints at obstruction of the small airways during acid perfusion of the esophagus. These changes were not produced in the control group: not in asthmatics with a sound esophagus and not in patients with sound lungs but a positive acid perfusion test of the esophagus (Fig. 2).

As the test was done in the upright position and no patient was coughing during the examination, aspiration does not seem to be the cause of the bronchial constriction. This reflex is probably a vagal reflex and may be initiated by esophageal irritation, esophageal dilatation or spasm. A retention of esophageal contents is propably not the cause, as demonstrated in one of our previous investigations (Kjellén 1981). In those studies asthmatic patients with dysfunction of the esophagus and the symptom of an "overloaded feeling" after meals were examined using scintigraphy. A retention of food after meals could not be found in the esophagus of these patients. The subjective feeling of overload is seen in many esophageal studies in patients with dysfunction of the esophagus. This symptom may be caused by delay of emptying of the stomach, which is often associated with GER.

Summarizing, I would like to stress that in all patients with asthma who do not respond to conventional therapy, esophageal dysfunction may be present and should be ruled out. First, one should ask the patient for esophageal symptoms. If necessary, roentgenography, manometry, acid perfusion test, acid clearance test, pH monitoring, and endoscopy are to be performed. The treatment of the esophageal dysfunction has an improving effect on the esophageal as well as on the bronchial symptoms.

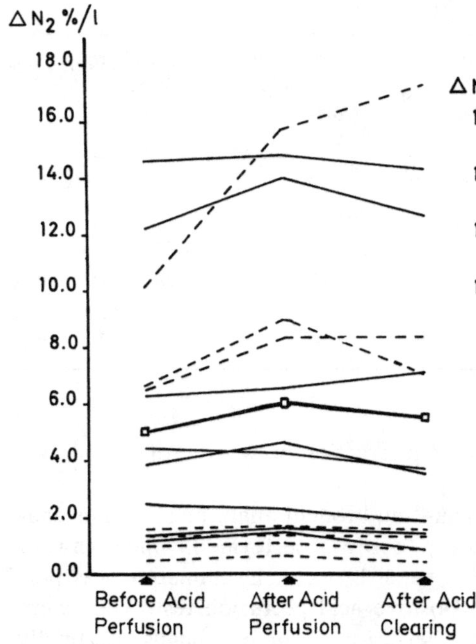

Fig. 1

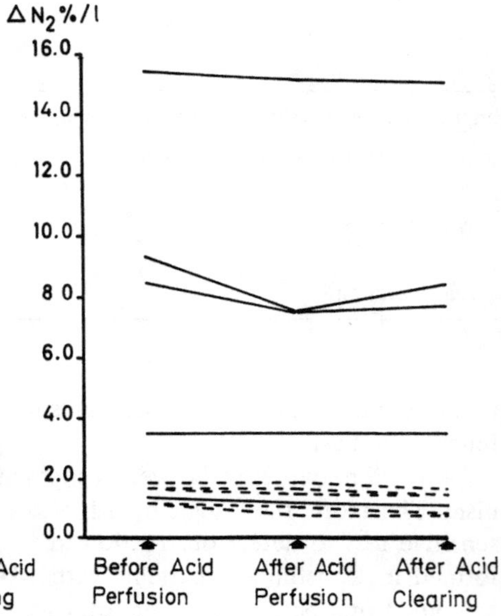

Fig. 2

Fig. 1. Inclination of the alveolar plateau ($\Delta N_2\%/1$) before and after acid perfusion and after acid clearing. --------, exogenous asthmatics; ————, endogenous asthmatics; □, mean in 15 asthmatics

Fig. 2. Inclination of the alveolar plateau ($\Delta N_2\%/1$) before and after acid perfusion and after acid clearing. --------, patients ($n = 5$) with normal lungs and a acid perfusion test; ————, asthmatics ($n = 5$) with negative acid perfusion test

Summary

In patients with asthma who do not respond to conventional therapy, esophageal dysfunction should be considered. The treatment of esophageal dysfunction has an improving effect on both the esophageal and the bronchial symptoms in these cases.

Résumé

Chez les malades atteints d'asthme qui ne répondent pas au traitement conventionnel, une dysfonction œsophagienne doit être suspectée. Le traitement de cette dysfonction a un effet bénéfique à la fois sur l'œsophage et sur les symptômes bronchiques dans ces cas.

Zusammenfassung

Bei Patienten mit Asthma, die nicht auf konventionelle Therapie ansprechen, muß eine Ösophagusdysfunktion in Betracht gezogen werden. Die Behandlung der Ösophagusdysfunktion bessert sowohl die Ösophagus- als auch die Asthmasymptome.

References

Fonkalsrud EW (1980) Gastroesophageal fundoplication for the management of chronic pulmonary disease in children. Am J Surg 140:72–79

Friedland GW, Yamate M, Marinkovich VA (1973) Hiatal hernia and chronic unremitting asthma. Pediatr Radiol 1:150–160

Ghaed N, Stein MR (1979) Assessment of a technique for scintigraphic monitoring of pulmonary aspiration of gastric contents in asthmatics with gastroesophageal reflux. Ann Allergy 42:306–308

Kjellén G (1981) Oesophageal dysfunction and bronchial asthma. Medical Dissertations, No. 111, Linköping University, Sweden

Mays EE (1976) Intrinsic asthma in adults. Association with gastroesophageal reflux. JAMA 236:2626–2628

Mendelson CL (1946) The aspiration of stomach contents into the lungs during obstetric anesthesia. Am J Obstet Gynecol 52:191–205

Mermod E (1887) Dilatation diffuse de l'oesophage sans rétrécissement organique. Rev Med Suisse Romande 7:422–424

Urschel HC, Paulson DL (1967) Gastroesophageal reflux and hiatal hernia. Complications and therapy. J Thorac Cardiovasc Surg 53:21–32

Esophageal and Pulmonary Scintiscanning in Gastroesophageal Reflux in Children

D. Berger[1], A. Bischof-Delaloye[2], O. Reinberg[1], and M. Roulet[3]

The clinical manifestations of gastroesophageal reflux (GER), according to Leape (1980), can be classified into three main syndromes: the general symptoms resulting from vomiting, the local and systemic effects of esophagitis, and, finally, the gastro-bronchopulmonary aspiration syndromes.

Over the past years, numerous authors (Gardy et al. 1982; Herbst et al. 1979; Herbst 1981; Ramenofsky and Leape 1981) have drawn attention to bronchopulmonary problems, particularly in the case of children who do not vomit. Subsequently, one may assume that pneumonia, atypical asthma crisis, neonatal apneic spells, chronic cough, and hoarseness can be attributed to GER and disappear if the reflux is treated conservatively or by surgery.

In 1976, Fisher et al. developed a method of scintiscanning to detect GER in adults. Since 1979, the first reports in infants and children have been published (Arasu et al. 1980; Blumhagen et al. 1980; Heyman et al. 1979; Rudd and Christie 1979). This examination allows the diagnosis of GER as well as the determination of its severity. In addition, it permits an appreciation of the esophageal dynamics (Heyman 1982) and, above all, gives definite proof of pulmonary aspiration of the gastric contents into the lungs (Chernow et al. 1979; Jona et al. 1981; Ramenofsky and Leape 1981).

Between December 1980 and December 1982, in Lausanne, we performed 19 scintiscans in order to detect a GER or a bronchopulmonary aspiration of gastric contents. In this paper, we analyze our own experience, compare it with that in the literature, and attempt to estimate the value of this diagnostic aid for the course of treatment applied.

Materials and Methods

Scintiscanning was carried out 19 times in 18 children (13 boys and five girls). The youngest, a former premature baby, was 5 mon old and the oldest was 12 years old. Eight children were under 1 year, and four were between 1 and 2 years old. All presented bronchopulmonary symptomatology, recurrent bronchopneumonia, atypical asthma, or apneic spells which could be attributed to a GER. In one child (No. 2), we suspected a syndrome of Sandifer (Leape 1980). In nine of these cases, vomiting was not the principal symptom (Table 1).

Services de chirurgie pédiatrique[1],
de médecine nucléaire[2] et
de pediatrie[3] du Centre Hospitalier Universitaire Vaudois (CHUV), CH-1011 Lausanne, Switzerland

Progress in Pediatric Surgery, Vol. 18
Ed. by P. Wurnig

Table 1. Clinical presentation and diagnostic tests in 18 children with suspected GER and pulmonary symptoms

			Symptoms		Endoscopy	Roentgenology	Scintiscan		
			Vomiting	Aspiration syndromes	Esophagitis	GER on BaGE	GER on RNGE	Disturbance in motility	Aspiration
1.	M.S.	5 y	–	+	–	–	–		–
2.	K.A.	8 m	–	+		+	+		–
3.	B.G.	10 m	+	+		–	–		–
4.	G.C.	8 m	–	+	–	–	–		–
5.	C.Th.	5 y	–	+		–	+		–
6.	H.M.	3 y	–	+		–	+		+
7.	D.G.	8 m	+	+	+	+	+	+	–
8.	G.O.	2 y	+	+	+	+	+	+	+
		2½ y	+	–		–	–	+	–
9.	I.A.	9 m	+	+		–	–	+	–
10.	N.M.	10 m	+	+		–	–	–	–
11.	R.L.	11 y	–	+	–	–	–		–
12.	G.P.	8 y	+	+	–	–	–		+
13.	T.C.	6 y	+	+		–	–	+	–
14.	K.A.	12 y	–	+		–	–	–	–
15.	S.A.	7 y	–	+		–	+	+	–
16.	R.Y.	5 m	+	Apneic spells		+	+	–	–
17.	B.M.	5 y	+	+		–	–	+	–
18.	I.J.	10 m	–	+		–	+	+	–

GER, gastroesophageal reflux
BaGE, barium gastroesophagography
RNGE, radionuclide gastroesophagography

The examination took place in the following manner. A nonreasonable radioactive tracer, technetium-99^{m} (^{99m}Tc sulfur colloid) is mixed with milk or fruit juice. The upper digestive tract is then "cleaned" by the same liquid without the tracer. For infants and small children, the absorbed volume is equivalent to a normal meal. The esophageal passage of the tracer is followed by a scintillation camera linked up with a computer. The "time-activity" curves of the upper, middle, and lower esophagus and of the stomach allow an appreciation of the esophageal dynamics, gastric drainage, and the presence of a GER (Heyman 1982; Leisner et al. 1982). In uncooperative infants and small children, the tracer is introduced directly into the stomach through a nasogastric tube to avoid aspiration while swallowing. Approximately 12 h later, normally the next morning, the presence of the tracer is looked for in the lungs, thereby proving a bronchial aspiration of the gastric contents during the preceeding hours (Heyman et al. 1979; Heyman 1982; Jona et al. 1981).

Results

The scintigraphy procedure has been somewhat modified during the last 2 years. In the beginning, we only studied signs of a bronchial aspiration of the tracer, then we demonstrated the presence and gravity of a GER, and finally we determined the esophageal dynamics.

Four patients with GER were discovered by upper gastrointestinal series and the gastroesophageal scintiscannings (Fig. 1). In four patients, the scintiscan

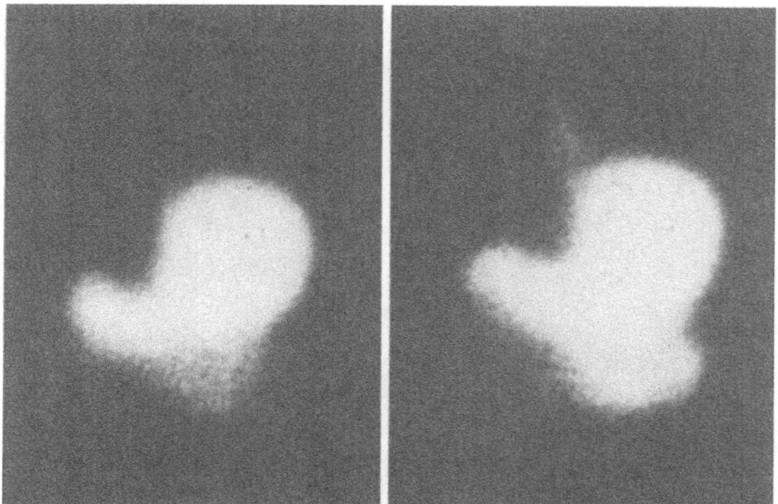

a b

Fig. 1. Positive GER after 15 s in a 2-year-old child (No. 8) with vomiting and recurrent pneumonia

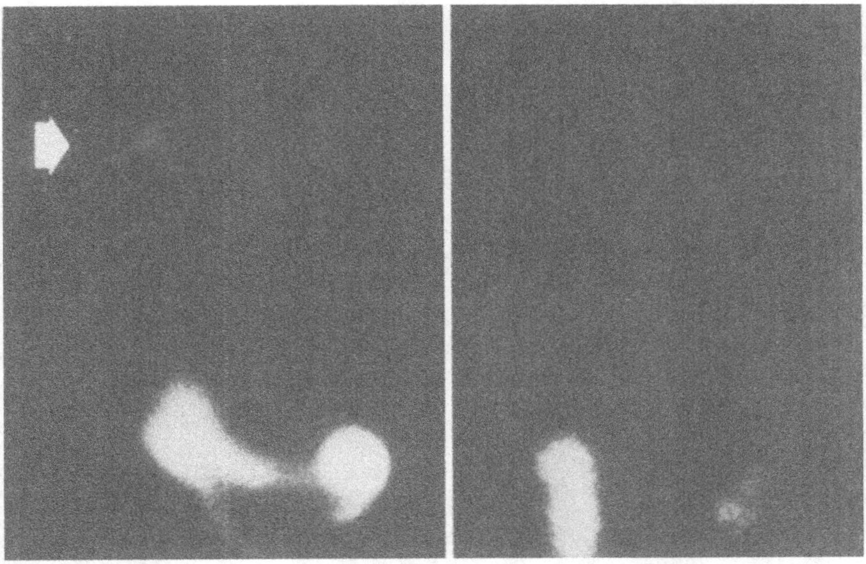

a b

Fig. 2. **a** Positive pulmonary scan *(arrow)* few hours later in the same child (No. 8). *Below,* normal activity in the colon. **b** Negative control 7 mon later after a Nissen operation

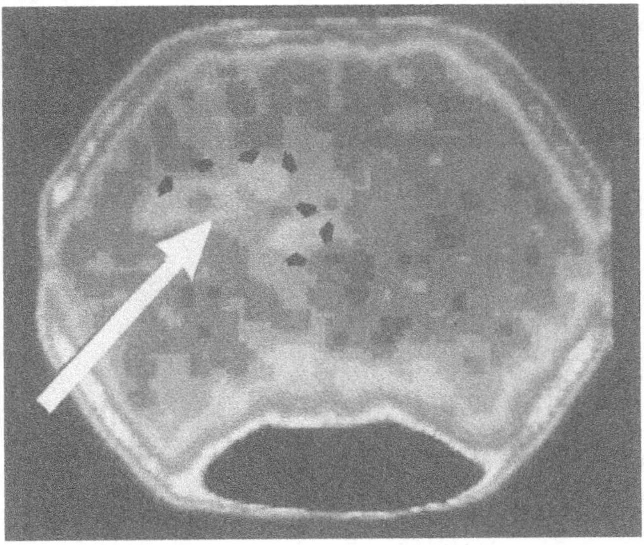

Fig. 3. A 3-year-old child (No. 6) with recurrent bronchitis and pneumonia. No GER either by upper gastrointestinal series or gastroesophageal scintiscanning, but positive pulmonary scan on the next day

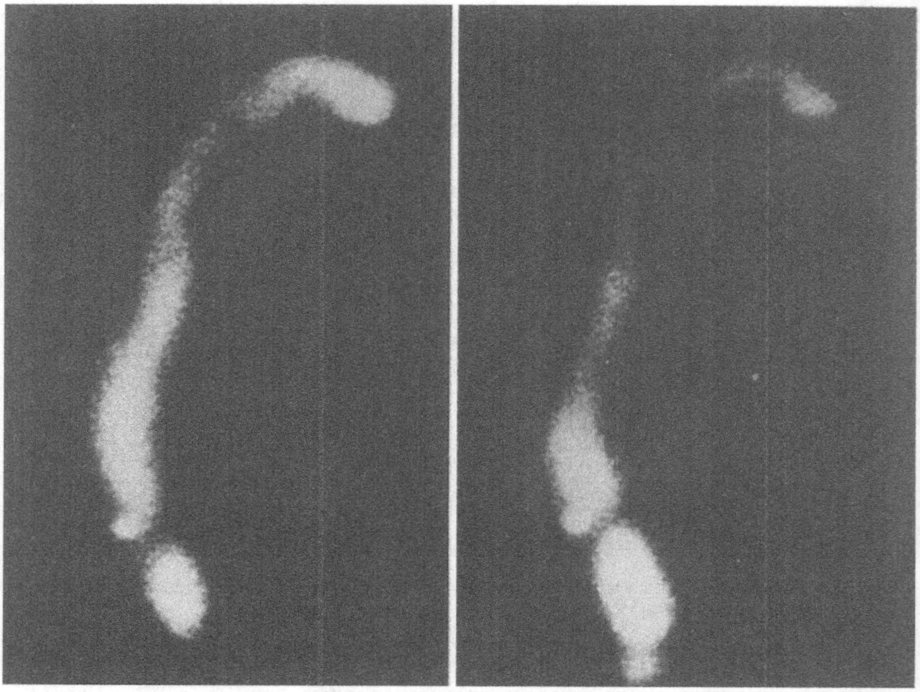

Fig. 4. Esophageal dyskinesia in an 8-year-old girl (No. 13) with recurrent pulmonary symptoms after operation for esophageal atresia

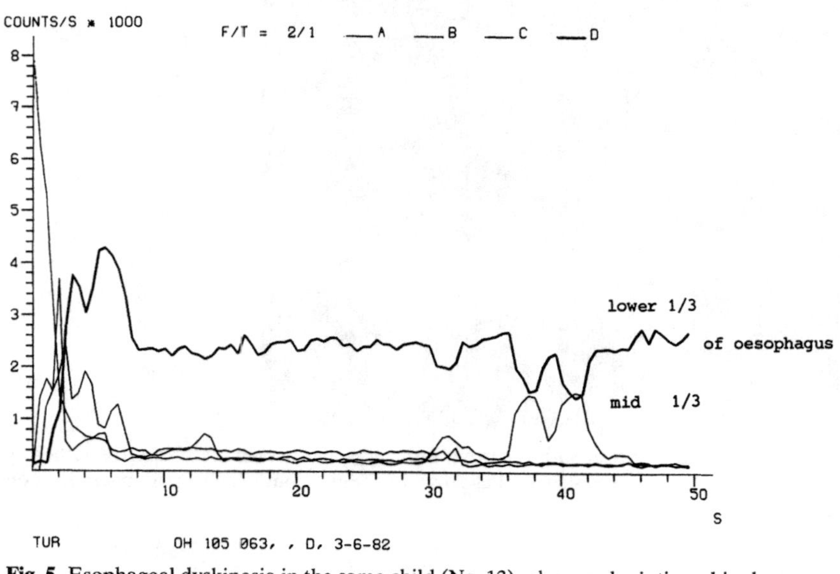

Fig. 5. Esophageal dyskinesia in the same child (No. 13): abnormal scintigraphic clearances of the mid and lower esophagus

showed a GER which was not seen on the roentgenographic examination. All the radiological GERs were also seen on scintiscan.

In three children, the pulmonary scan was positive (Figs. 2, 3). One of them (No. 12) had no GER, either on the upper gastrointestinal series or on the scintiscan half an hour later (Fig. 4). Eight cases of esophageal dyskinesia were observed (Fig. 5); four were associated with GER and two followed Nissen's operation (Nos. 8 and 13). Only one of these children had esophagitis on endoscopy (No. 8).

Discussion

The esophageal and pulmonary scintiscan is a simple technique, permitting detection of a GER (Arasu et al. 1980; Blumhagen et al. 1980; Fisher et al. 1976; Heyman et al. 1979; Jona et al. 1981; Piepsz et al. 1981; Rudd and Christie 1979). This examination is two to three times more precise than a barium gastroesophagography (Table 2). Only Blumhagen et al. in 1980 discovered more radiological GERs (74% against 63%) by using the "water siphon test" during radiological transit. In our study, the scintiscan demonstrated a reflux in four instances when none was demonstrated roentgenographically.

The examination takes place under more physiological conditions than the radiological investigation, even permitting the infants to sleep. It can be prolonged when wished and can indicate an intermittent GER. It is, however, less sensitive than long-term esophageal pH monitoring (Herbst 1981; Leape 1980).

Table 2. Demonstration of gastroesophgeal reflux

	Patients (*n*)	Positive RNGE (%)	Positive BaGE (%)
Fisher 1976	30	90	60
Rudd 1979	25	80	60
Heyman 1979	39	59	26
Arasu 1980	30	57	50
Blumhagen 1980	65	63	74[a]
Jona 1981	125	77	55
Piepsz 1981	24	67	79[b]
CHUV 1982	18	44	22

RNGE, radionuclide gastroesophagography
BaGE, barium gastroesophagography

[a] Water siphon test by BaGE
[b] RNGE four times. On roentgenogram, reflux grade 1 (water siphon test)

Table 3. Demonstration of aspiration using pulmonary scintiscanning

	Patients (*n*)	GER on BaGE	Positive pulmonary scintiscan	
Reich 1977	7		2	Adults
Chernow 1979	5		2	Adults
Heyman 1979	39	10	2	21 reflux on RNGE
Arasu 1980	30	15	0[a]	
Blumhagen 1980	10	10	0	96 reflux on RNGE
Jona 1980	125	38	18	
Piepsz 1981	35		0	
CHUV 1982	16	4	3	8 reflux on RNGE

[a] Negative in spite of clinical evidence of pulmonary aspiration of gastric contents in two patients
RNGE, radionuclide gastroesophagography
BaGE, barium gastroesophagography
GER, gastroesophageal reflux

Pulmonary scintiscanning, performed several hours later or the following day, is at present the only method of demonstrating bronchial aspiration of gastric origin (Chernow et al. 1979; Heyman et al. 1979; Jona et al. 1981; Reich et al. 1977). On three occasions, we were able to determine its existence and to control the symptomatology (one Nissen's operation and two medical treatments) (Table 3). There does not exist, as yet, a comparative study between upper esophageal pH monitoring (Ramenofsky and Leape 1981) and pulmonary scintiscanning. It may be possible that different timing or a repetition of the examination would allow us to discover more pulmonary involvement especially in children presenting evidence of aspiration (Arasu et al. 1980) (Table 3).

Another advantage of the scintiscan is the reduced radiation exposure. Fisher et al. (1976) reports that it is 30 times less than in radiological examination – at least in the esophageal region. However, it is slightly less favorable if intestinal transit is slowed down and more acceptable when compared with radiological examination requiring a prolonged fluoroscopy (Blumhagen et al. 1980; Heyman 1982; Piepsz et al. 1981; Rudd and Christie 1979). Leape (1980) thinks that the radiation dose is negligible.

On the other hand, it is difficult to compare the esophagoscopy and the scintiscan. Endoscopy is rarely a first choice examination. It is the only one which can indicate the gravity of an esophagitis.

The first results in the literature and our own experience are encouraging. The esophageal and pulmonary scintiscan in the diagnosis of a GER is a noninvasive method, allowing a continuous or repetitive observation. In addition, it is more precise than an upper gastrointestinal series, while giving the patient a lower dose of radiation.

In conclusion, which examination should be chosen if a GER is suspected (Table 4)? The decision depends on the symptomatology and the gravity of one

Table 4. Comparison between scintiscanning and other diagnostic procedures to detect GER in children

Radionuclide gastroesophagography with lung scintiscanning

Compared with	Advantage	Disadvantage
Barium gastro-esophagography	– More sensitive – More physiological – Lower radiation exposure – Intermittent episodes of GER may be seen – Aspiration during bed rest or sleep may be proved	– No morphological study – Dynamic: less qualitative
pH Monitoring	– No delicate esophageal catheter – Shorter examination	– Quantitatively less precise – Less sensitive for demonstration of intermittent episodes of GER
Endoscopy	– No narcosis	– No morphological study (esophagitis)

GER, gastroesophageal reflux

of the three syndromes of Leape (1980). If chronic vomiting predominates, especially in infants, the upper gastrointestinal series with morphological and dynamic studies is the best choice (syndrome of Roviralta, hiatus hernia). On the other hand, when esophagitis is suspected (dysphagia, discomfort after feeding, heartburn, awakening from sleep in pain with or without vomiting, macroscopic or occult blood in vomit or in stools, low hemoglobin, etc.), the roentgenogram, rapidly followed by endoscopy of the esophagus, stomach, and duodenum, is by far preferable. They allow appreciation of the gravity of the inflammatory lesions or their scars. Esophageal manometry, useful in studying physiopathology, is only exceptionally recommended as a diagnostic method.

Finally, all the other presentations of GER, with or without vomiting (Leape 1980; Weissbluth 1981), motivate an esophageal and pulmonary scintiscan. Its use is more simple than pH monitoring (Arasu et al. 1980; Gardy et al. 1982; Leape 1980; Ramenofsky and Leape 1981). This investigation is shorter and almost as sensitive.

In this manner, the scintiscanning of the esophagus and the lungs should in the future be the first examination to be undertaken when the pulmonary aspiration of gastric contents is suspected.

Summary

The analysis of 19 esophageal and pulmonary scintiscans performed with a non-reabsorbable radioactive tracer shows that this is a simple and efficient way of detecting the presence of a GER or a bronchial aspiration of gastric contents in children. This examination proves to be more sensitive, with a lower amount of radiation necessary, than the radiological gastroesophagography. It is less invasive and takes place under more physiological conditions. It is especially useful when symptoms lead one to suspect a syndrome of GER with aspiration.

Résumé

L'analyse de 19 scintigraphies œsophagiennes et pulmonaires chez l'enfant, à l'aide d'un traceur radioactif non-résorbable, montre qu'il s'agit d'un moyen simple et efficace pour détecter la présence de reflux gastro-œsophagien ou d'une broncho-aspiration du contenu gastrique. Cet examen s'est révélé plus sensible et moins irradiant que la transit gastro-œsophagien radiologique. Il est moins invasif et se déroule dans des conditions plus physiologiques. Il est surtout utile en face d'un examen clinique faisant suspecter un syndrome d'aspiration secondaire d'un reflux gastro-œsophagien.

Zusammenfassung

Die Analyse von 19 Lungen- und Ösophagusszintigraphien bei Kindern mit Hilfe eines nichtresorbierbaren radioaktiven Trägers (^{99m}Tc) zeigt, daß es sich hierbei um eine einfache und zuverlässige Untersuchungsmethode handelt, um einen gastroösophagealen Reflux oder eine Aspiration des Mageninhalts zu diagnostizieren. Diese Untersuchung ist genauer als eine röntgenologische Ösophagus-Magen-Passage und die Strahlenbelastung ist wesentlich geringer. Sie ist nicht invasiv und wird unter physiologischeren Bedingungen durchgeführt. Sie ist besonders nützlich beim klinischen Verdacht eines sekundären, durch gastroösophagealen Reflux hervorgerufenen Aspirationssyndroms.

References

Arasu TS, Wyllie R, Fitzgerald JF, Franken EA, Siddiqui AR, Lehman GA, Eigen H, Grosfeld JL (1980) Gastroesophageal reflux in infants and children. Comparative accuracy of diagnostic methods. J Pediatr 96:798–803

Blumhagen JD, Rudd TG, Christie DL (1980) Gastroesophageal reflux in children: radionuclide gastroesophagography. AJR 135:1001–1004

Chernow B, Johson LF, Janowitz WR, Castell DO (1979) Pulmonary aspiration as a consequence of gastroesophageal reflux. Dig Dis Sci 24:839–844

Fisher RS, Malmund LS (1981) Esophageal scintigraphy: are there advantages? Gastroenterology 80:1066–1067

Fisher RS, Malmund LS, Roberts GS, Lobis IF (1976) Gastroesophageal (GE) scintiscanning to detect and quantitate GE reflux. Gastroenterology 70:301–308

Gardy J, Arana J, Alzueta M, Zaldwa J, Tovar J (1982) Le reflux gastro-oesophagien à manifestations respiratoires. Helv Paediatr Acta 37:221–230

Herbst JJ (1981) Gastroesophageal reflux. J Pediatr 98:859–870

Herbst JJ, Minton SD, Book LS (1979) Gastroesophageal reflux causing respiratory distress and apnea in newborn infants. J Pediatr 95:763–768

Heyman S (1982) Esophageal scintigraphy (milk scans) in infants and children with gastroesophageal reflux. Radiology 144:881–893

Heyman S, Kirkpatrick JA, Winter HS, Treves S (1979) An improved radionuclide method for the diagnosis of gastroesophageal reflux and aspiration in children (milk scan). Radiology 131:479–482

Jona JZ, Sty JR, Glicklich M (1981) Simplified radioisotope technique for assessing gastroesophageal reflux in children. J Pediatr Surg 16:114–117

Leape LL (1980) Gastroesophageal reflux. In: Holder TM, Ashcraft RW (eds) Pediatric surgery, chap 24. Saunders, Philadelphia, pp 292–312

Leisner B, Wirsching R, Seidl I (1982) Ösophagus-Funktions-Szintigraphie: Kombinierte Untersuchung von Peristaltik und gastroösophagealem Reflux. Nucl Compact 13:188–194

Piepsz A, Georges B, Perlmutter N, Rodesch P, Cadramel S (1981) Gastroesophageal scintiscanning in children. Pediatr Radiol 11:71–74

Ramenofsky ML, Leape LL (1981) Continous upper esophageal pH monitoring in infants and children with gastroesophageal reflux, pneumonia, and apneic spells. J Pediatr Surg 16: 374–378

Reich SB, Earley WC, Ravin TH, Goodman M, Spector S, Stein MR (1977) Evaluation of gastro-pulmonary aspiration by a radioactive technique: concise communication. J Nucl Med 18:1079–1081

Rudd TG, Christie DL (1979) Demonstration of gastroesophageal reflux in children by radionuclide gastroesophagography. Radiology 131:483–486

Weissbluth M (1981) Gastroesophageal reflux: a review. Clin Pediatr 20:7–14

Conservative Treatment of Gastroesophageal Reflux and Hiatus Hernia

J. P. GUGGENBICHLER and G. MENARDI[1]

Introduction

Few disorders have been the center of so much controversy over the last 10 years as gastroesophageal reflux (GER) and hiatus hernia. There have been widespread differences in the assessment of its etiology, pathophysiology, incidence, and significance. When GER is established as the cause of the patient's symptoms, there is far from uniform agreement as to the best mode of therapy and the indication for surgical treatment.

As evidence accumulates it has become apparent that GER is a common problem, particularly in young infants. GER is the regurgitation of gastric contents into the esophagus and even into the pharynx. GER, while usually associated with hiatus hernia, may occur also in the absence of any demonstrable anatomic malformation.

From a pediatric point of view, we consider GER as the main symptom of lower esophageal sphincter incompetence. A classification of these disturbances of the lower esophagus is offered by Schäfer (1967): this also suits best our opinion about the pathophysiology of this disorder.

Classification of Disturbances of the Lower Esophagus

Malfunction

Normally the lower esophageal sphincter (LES) is closed and opens upon arrival of esophageal peristalsis. The coordination of esophageal peristalsis and opening and closure of the LES, however, is immature during the first 4–6 weeks of life. The great majority of children vomit as their sole symptom, particularly when placed in the left recumbent position. Chalasia is a transient relaxation of the LES and esophagus as a whole. Differentiation of chalasia from peristaltic disarrangement and from *formes mineures* of hiatus hernia is impossible on clinical grounds.

Malposition

The presence of an intraabdominal segment of esophagus and the acute angle of the entry of the esophagus into the stomach presumably contribute to prevention

[1] Department of Pediatric Surgery, University of Innsbruck, Anichstr. 35, A-6020 Innsbruck/Austria

Progress in Pediatric Surgery, Vol. 18
Ed. by P. Wurnig

of reflux in normal children. The obliteration of these two factors by hiatus hernia may partially explain the frequent association of reflux and hiatus hernia. In hiatus hernia the LES slides upward into the thoracic cavity and pulls a portion of stomach with it. The reason for this displacement of the LES is a poor fixation of the cardia and esophagus by the phrenicoesophageal membrane and the abdominal mesoesophagus.

Severe and prolonged reflux and vomiting is seen with sliding hiatus hernia and may lead to secondary, life-threatening complications.

Growth failure is very common. Peptic esophagitis from constant reflux of gastric acid may cause gastrointestinal bleeding, anemia, and severe iron depletion. Continued esophagitis eventually leads to transmural esophageal stricture and progressive dysphagia.

Brachyesophagus

Brachyesophagus, considered by many authors as a consequence of peptic esophagitis, is, according to our opinion, a primary malformation, and not a secondary event.

Incidence and Clinical Manifestations

Gastroesophageal incompetence and vomiting are frequent occurrences in pediatric patients. Between 1975 and 1982, a total of 102 children were admitted to our clinics with persistent vomiting. Of these, 67 children were diagnosed as having atonic vomiting or chalasia. The true incidence of this problem is probably much higher, as parents and physicians tend to start appropriate therapy without prior diagnostic measures once history and physical examination suggest GER. Within a matter of a few weeks of postural and dietary therapy, symptoms subside in the patients with functional problems and relatively few children are referred for further evaluation of persistent symptoms. Hiatus hernia was observed in 35 children during the same period of time. There were 22 infants below the age of 1 year, and 13 children beyond 1 year. The percentage of mentally retarded children among the 13 older patients was remarkably high.

All children with radiographically proven hiatus hernia showed persistent – frequently bloodstained – vomiting, malnutrition, bloody stools, and severe iron deficiency anemia.

Serious pulmonary complications, which are most emphasized in the literature, were observed only once in the workup of children with recurrent pneumonias and the near miss sudden infant death syndrome despite a constant awareness of this complication.

Our conception about the physiology of the lower esophageal sphincter, the pathophysiology of sphincter incompetence, and GER is followed by a strong belief that almost all children with LES incompetence and hiatus hernia, even with the serious complication of peptic reflux esophagitis, can be treated by conservative means.

The central idea behind this is: Children tend to grow out of it!

With maturation, dietary changes, and assumption of the upright position, reflux tends to disappear.

By the time they reach the age of 12–15 mon, 90% of children with symptoms of reflux will be free of symptoms.

Clearly any therapeutic intervention should be designed with this in mind!

The most important therapeutic measure is postural therapy. If symptoms are mild, placement of the patient in an infant chair for an hour or so after feeding may be all that is required. With more severe symptoms, it may be necessary to maintain the patient in an upright position 24 hours a day. The seat should be properly padded and the child be strapped in to prevent him or her from falling forward or slouching. Propping the child up with pillows is ineffective in these severe cases.

Duration of therapy is usually several weeks to months, and usually for an additional 6 weeks after symptoms have subsided and the patient has started to gain weight. These therapeutic measures were sufficient for 19 infants out of 22 (86.3%). Among these successfully treated patients was also one 5-mon-old infant with a gastroscopically proven peptic esophagitis. Three children had to be operated upon during this period of time.

For treatment of peptic reflux esophagitis, review of the relevant literature revealed several additional therapeutic measures upon which I will comment.

Postural therapy

Thickening of formula with cereal (1 tablespoon/60 ml)

Reduction of volume of feeding; increasing the frequency

Medication
- Antacids
- Cimetidine
- Metoclopramide
- Local anesthetics
- Carbenoxolone
- Bethanechol

It is our firm belief that postural therapy and the administration of frequent, small feedings is all that is necessary. Thickening of feedings we consider useless. The administration of an adapted infant formula (Hippon A, NAN, Preaptamil) ensures optimal growth and gain of weight. In our hands, formula was never thickened and we were able to achieve our therapeutic success without this measure.

Drug therapy is also controversial. Metoclopramide has serious side effects if one exceeds the therapeutic range. Handling of this drug in children is quite difficult. Therefore, we consider this drug as contraindicated. Carbenoxolone has, besides a questionable efficacy, serious side effects (aldosterone-simulating mode of action).

Bethanechol has parasympathomimetic effects on the gastrointestinal tract with hydrochloric acid production, cramping abdominal pain, and diarrhea. This drug, although recommended in Anglo-American literature, is not available in central Europe.

The most important aspect of therapy is: careful feeding – frequent, small feedings – and postural therapy. Peptic reflux esophagitis can be treated for the first 8–10 days with cimetidine, although pediatric experience with this drug is rather scarce. There is no experience with this drug for long-term therapy.

Surgical intervention is indicated in a child that doesn't respond to careful conservative therapy and presents symptoms beyond the time at which the patient may be expected to grow out of reflux (usually 12–15 months). Surgical treatment is indicated earlier if the symptoms are uncontrollable and are disabling or life endangering (such as failure to thrive that is refractory to medical treatment over a 2–3 months period, serious pulmonary complications, and a history of near miss sudden infant death).

Immediate surgical treatment is indicated for patients with strictures and congenital brachyesophagus.

Older children with significant symptoms from GER should also be considered for surgical therapy, especially in the case of retarded children.

Summary

Gastroesophageal reflux is a frequent occurrence in infancy. Most frequently, gastroesophageal reflux (GER) is due to a functional disturbance and lack of coordination of esophageal motility and lower esophageal sphincter incompetence. Vomiting is the sole symptom in the great majority of infants and responds readily to postural and dietary therapy.

A malposition and defective fixation of the cardia and abdominal esophagus is the pathophysiologic substrate of hiatus hernia. Although most patients with hiatus hernia have GER, hiatus hernia is only symptomatic with concomitant GER. Differentiation between hiatus hernia and GER should therefore be dispelled.

Treatment of hiatus hernia with GER is directed towards placing the patient in an upright position, even 24 h a day if necessary in a patient severe symptoms. The duration of therapy can be weeks to months. Small, frequent feedings are of additional importance, while thickening of formula with cereals were found unnecessary.

Over the last few years, we have been able to observe 22 infants under 1 year of age with GER and hiatus hernia. In 19 of these patients – among them also patients with reflux esophagitis – this conservative treatment regimen has been successful. Drugs like antacids or cimetidine to lower gastric were considered unnecessary. Bethanechol was considered contra-indicated due to its discomforting side effects in infants. Three patients have been treated surgically during this period of time.

In contrast, hiatus hernia in older children – mainly mentally retarded children – with GER has to be treated surgically; conservative therapy is usually without effect.

The rare clinical condition of brachyesophagus is considered a malformation and requires surgical therapy in every instance.

Résumé

Le reflux gastro-œsophagien est fréquent chez les nourrissons. Il s'agit le plus souvent d'une dysfonction liée à un manque de coordination entre cardia et péristaltisme. La chalasie est un relâchement passager du cardia et de l'œsophage et est, en général, très facile à traiter: position assise, repas fréquents et légers y mettent fin en l'espace de quelques semaines.

Par contre, nous considérons la hernie hiatale comme une perturbation positionnelle, due à une malfixation du cardia et de l'œsophage abdominal. Durant les 5 dernières années, nous avons observé 22 nourrissons présentant une hernie hiatale par glissement et un reflux gastro-œsophagien. 19 nourrissons furent maintenus en position assise ininterrompue, pendant des semaines, voire des mois dans les cas particulièrement graves. Les repas étaient fréquents et légers et il ne nous a pas semblé utile d'épaissir les aliments. Les résultats thérapeutiques nous ont par la suite donné raison. Nous n'avons pas non plus administré de médicaments, même dans les cas d'œsophagie par reflux associé, ni anti-acides, ni cimétédine, ni paspertine, ni béthanéchol bien qu'ils soient recommandés dans la littérature. 3 nourrissons seulement ont dû être opérés pendant l'étude.

Par contre, nous avons observé et opéré immédiatement 13 enfants, mentalement handicapés le plus souvent, et présentant une hernie du hiatus et un reflux œsophagien.

Quant au brachyœsophage, assez rare, nous le considérons comme une malformation à opérer sans exception.

Zusammenfassung

Der gastroösophageale Reflux ist ein häufiges Ereignis im Säuglingsalter. Am häufigsten findet er sich als funktionale Störung des Zusammenspiels von Kardia und Ösophagusmotorik. Die Chalasie ist ein passageres Erschlaffen von Kardia und Ösophagus und erfordert meist nur Hochlagerung und häufigere kleine Mahlzeiten. Der therapeutische Erfolg stellt sich meist bereits nach wenigen Wochen ein.

Demgegenüber betrachten wir die gleitende Hiatushernie als eine Lagestörung, als deren Ursache eine Störung der Fixation der Kardia und des Ösophagus abdominalis angesehen wird.

Wir konnten in den letzten 5 Jahren 22 Säuglinge mit einer gleitenden Hiatushernie und gastroösophagealem Reflux an unserer Klinik beobachten. 19 Säuglinge wurden konservativ mit Hochlagerung – in schweren Fällen ununterbrochen über Wochen bzw. Monate – und häufigen kleinen Mahlzeiten behandelt. Eine Eindickung der Nahrung wurde nicht durchgeführt bzw. als nicht nötig erachtet, wobei uns die therapeutischen Resultate recht geben.

Eine medikamentöse Therapie wurde ebenso nicht durchgeführt, auch nicht bei begleitender Refluxösophagitis.

Antacida, Cimetidin, Paspertin und Bethanechol, wie sie in der Literatur empfohlen werden, wurden bei keinem Patienten verabreicht.

Nur 3 Säuglinge wurden im selben Zeitraum operiert. Demgegenüber wurden 13 ältere Kinder, meist geistig behinderte, mit Hiatushernie und Reflux beobachtet und sofort einer chirurgischen Behandlung zugeführt.

Der seltene Brachyösophagus wird als Mißbildung betrachtet und wird ebenso immer chirurgisch behandelt.

References

Behar J, Sheahan DG, Brianconi P, Spiro HM (1975) Medical and surgical management of reflux esophagitis. A 38 month report on a prospective clinical trial. N Engl J Med 293:263–265

Darling DB, Fisher JH, Gellis SS (1974) Hiatal hernia and gastroesophageal reflux in infants and children: analysis of the incidence in North American children. Pediatrics 56:450–456

Koch A, Kehrer B, Bettex M (1982) Zur Operationsindikation bei der Kardiainsuffizienz des Säuglings. (Indication for surgical treatment of gastrooesophageal reflux in infants.) Z Kinderchir 36:146–150

Leape L (1982) Gastrooesophageal reflux and hiatal hernia. Curr Pediatr Ther 10:165–168

Neff G (1980) Gastroösophagealer Reflux. Schweizerischer Chirurgenkongreß, 1980, Lausanne

Schäfer KH (1967) Erkrankungen des Magendarmkanals. Angeborene Störungen der Cardia. In: Fanconi G, Wallgren A (Hrsg) Lehrbuch der Pädiatrie. Schwabe, Basel Stuttgart, S 736–739

Sonnenberg A, Giger M, Blum AL (1979) Behandlung des gastro-oesophagealen Reflux. Acta Gastroligie 8(3):261–275

Gastroesophageal Reflux and Severe Mental Retardation

A. F. Schärli[1]

Recurrent vomiting is very common in children with severe mental retardation. Nutritional deficiencies, anemia, and repeated bouts of aspiration pneumonitis impede the physical development of these children who already have motor defects. Often, this vomiting is written off as psychogenic, and a variety of methods are employed in attempts to overcome it, including antiemetic drugs, punishment, or a permanent nasogastric tube.

In many of these cases, thorough investigation reveals incompetence of the gastroesophageal sphincter or a hiatus hernia.

Our Own Patient Population

The analysis of our own patient population (Schaerli and Rumlova 1980) prompted us to distinguish between primary congenital gastroesophageal reflux and secondary reflux which is acquired in the course of infancy or early childhood

Table 1. Symptoms according to the various causes of gastroesophageal reflux in 50 operated children

Indication for antireflux surgery	*n*	Symptoms				
		Vomiting	Weight <3%ile	Esophagitis	Stenosis	Respiratory disturbance
Primary GER	31	31	12	17	2	13
Secondary GER	19					
– Mental retardation	10	10	4	6	2	5
– Esophageal anomaly	3	3	1	0	0	2
– Pyloric abstruction	2	2	2	2	0	0
– Secondary damage to hiatus	4	4	1	0	0	1
Total	50	50	20	25	4	21

[1]Department of Pediatric Surgery, Children's Hospital Lucerne, CH-6000 Luzern/Switzerland

Progress in Pediatric Surgery, Vol. 18
Ed. by P. Wurnig

(Table 1). Of those with secondary forms, children with severe mental retardation are affected most frequently, comprising 20% of all cases operated upon at our institution. Three of these required surgery during the 1st year of life and seven were operated upon between 4 and 16 years of age.

Symptoms

It is our impression that the clinical symptoms are particularly important. In all patients, the most prominent symptom was therapy-resistent vomiting, which was frequently characterized as rumination. It occurred at any time: during, after, or long after eating. It was not influenced by food consistency: normal, purée, or liquid feedings. It had nearly always been present since infancy or early childhood. Four children were severely malnourished due to the vomiting, and their weights were well below the third percentile at the time of examination. In six cases there had been repeated hematemesis or vomiting of coffee-ground material. Five children had had recurrent episodes of bronchitis or bronchopneumonia. Three children had reflux-induced laryngospasm which was occasionally followed by apnea. One of these children died of an irreversible cardiac arrest secondary to massive aspiration before permission to perform an antireflux operation had been obtained.

Physically, nearly all the children were delicate and bedridden; none was able to walk. None had an IQ over 60.

Workup

These children had obligatory gastroesophageal reflux, mainly in the form of chalasia of the cardia.

Two patients already had severe esophageal stenosis (Fig. 1). In six children, there was substantial erosive esophagitis. In two children, the diagnosis of a protein-losing enteropathy had previously been made, two had been diagnosed as having Herter's syndrome, and one had a disaccharidase deficiency. In two children, the X-ray study had to be discontinued prematurely due to massive aspiration of the contrast medium (Fig. 2).

Results

Ten children were treated by Nissen's fundoplication. In all cases, the postoperative course was favorable. The stenoses were relieved by repeated bougienage. Children who had previously appeared to ruminate were now capable of normal food intake. Weight gains were apparent within a few weeks. In five children, highly significant psychomotor advances were achieved within 6 mon. Two boys, who had been bedridden for 12 years, learned to walk almost without assistance

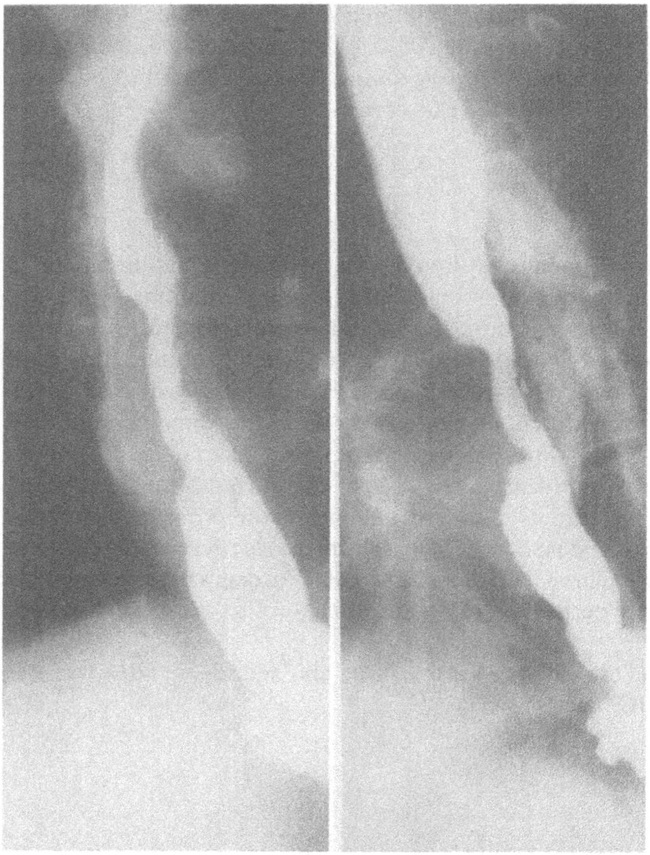

Fig. 1. Gastroesophageal reflux with severe esophageal stenosis in a 14-year-old boy with severe mental retardation; he was also bedridden and dystrophic

within 1 year. With a number of children there was a definite impression that verbal comprehension or their mode of expression had improved substantially since their nourishment had improved. The supposed disorders of bowel function (Herter's syndrome, protein-losing enteropathy, and disaccharidase deficiency), which had been diagnosed in five children, were seen to no longer be present postoperatively. These changes were apparent within days to weeks after the nutritional capacity improved.

Discussion

Little is written about the coincidence of mental retardation and gastroesophageal reflux. Abrahams and Burkett (1970) found hiatus hernias in 27% of 63 children

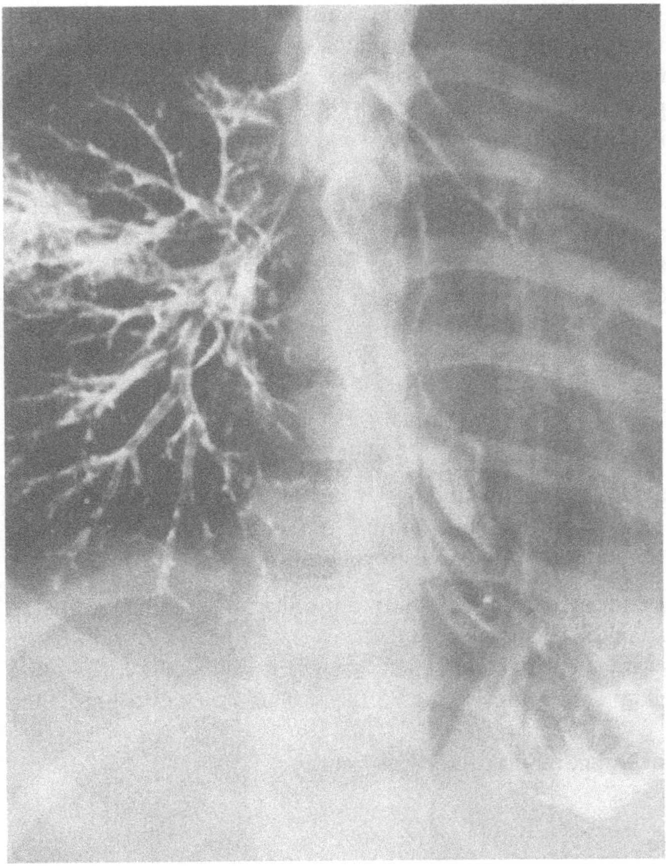

Fig. 2. Gastroesophageal reflux and cricopharyngeal spasm in a 7-year-old girl with hydrocephalus. Immediate aspiration on attempting to drink. Repeated episodes of apnea

with severe spasticity. Holmes (1971) reported that hiatus hernia was present in nearly all of 103 patients with spastic paraplegia and vomiting. In Johnson's series of 55 children with gastroesophageal reflux, eight were mentally retarded (Johnson et al. 1977).

Etiology

The etiological connection between gastroesophageal reflux and severe mental retardation cannot be directly explained. Holmes (1971) believes that excessive parasympathetic activity is responsible for chronically lowering the tone of the cardiac sphincter.

By clinical observation and manometric studies, Höllwarth and Sauer (1979) repeatedly observed attacks of apnea associated with gastroesophageal reflux, which implies some cerebral dysfunction. The constant supine position of the children with cerebral damage also appears to play a significant role in the occurrence of gastroesophageal reflux. In addition, the permanent spasticity of the abdominal wall, and probably also the diaphragm, is of importance.

Poor coordination of the swallowing mechanism due to vagal dysfunction must also be considered.

Manometric studies by Sondheimer and Morris (1979) revealed cardiac sphincter pressures of less than 10 mmHg in all these children. Our own studies failed to confirm this constancy. However, we repeatedly found evidence that vomiting became intensified in direct association with spasms of the abdominal muscles.

Indications for Operative Therapy

In mentally normal children, the indication for surgery is based *clinically* on the vomiting, *endoscopically* on the findings of esophagitis and stenosis, and *radiologically* on the chalasia or the hiatus hernia. In mentally retarded children, a number of additional symptoms come into consideration.

- Marked dysphagia and increasing irritability not only indicate uncoordinated peristalsis but also pain on swallowing.
- Spasms, which represent episodes of reflux, are often followed by aspiration and associated with apnea, cyanosis, and stiffness. This series of events is life threatening.
- The same is true for reflux-induced laryngospasm.

Choice of Procedure

Despite our reservations regarding Nissen's fundoplication, we have selected this procedure for all mentally retarded children. The absolute freedom from reflux outweighs the disadvantages of fundoplication in patients with spasms of the abdominal muscles and diaphragm who are constantly in the supine position.

Conclusions

Several conclusions may be drawn from the observations on gastroesophageal reflux in patients with severe mental retardation discussed above.

- It is desirable to position the bedridden children with the head somewhat elevated or to get them up at a standing board or into a standing apparatus intermittently.
- Repeated vomiting necessitates the early administration of antacids (or cimetidine), since these children are prone to develop esophagitis and esophageal stenosis.

- Mentally retarded children who vomit should have a barium swallow and esophagoscopy as soon as possible. Fundoplication should be performed before complications develop.
- Spasms and aspiration followed by apnea are life-threatening situations. Surgery is absolutely indicated in these cases.
- Physical dystrophy, malnutrition, and faulty development can often be prevented by an effective antireflux mechanism, and mental development can be promoted by operative therapy.

Summary

Recurrent vomiting is common in children with severe mental retardation and leads to significant morbidity with malnutrition, anemia, and aspiration pneumonitis. Spasms of the abdominal muscles and diaphragm, uncoordinated peristalsis, and central nervous system disorders are causes of dysphagia and continuous gastroesophageal reflux.

It is desirable that mentally retarded children with vomiting have a barium swallow and esophagoscopy as early as possible. Fundoplication should be performed before complications develop. Spasms with aspiration followed by apnea, in particular, are life-threatening situations. After surgery there is a definite improvement in mental and physical development.

Résumé

Les vomissements récidivants sont fréquents chez les enfants mentalement handicapés et comportent une morbidité significative par malnutrition, anémie, et pneumonie par aspiration. Les spasmes des muscles abdominaux et du diaphragme, le péristaltisme mal coordonné, et les désordres du système nerveux central sont des causes de dysphagie et de reflux gastro-œsophagien continuel. Il est souhaitable que les enfants mentalement retardés subissent un examen baryté et un œsophagoscopie aussitôt que possible. Une fundoplication doit être pratiquée avant que les complications ne se développent. Les spasmes avec aspiration alimentaire suivis d'apnée, peuvent avoir des conséquences mortelles. Après intervention chirurgicale on note une nette amélioration de l'état mental et physique de l'enfant.

Zusammenfassung

Rezidivierendes Erbrechen ist häufig bei Kindern mit schwerer geistiger Behinderung und führt zu erheblichen Krankheitserscheinungen mit Unterernährung,

Anämie und Aspirationspneumonie. Spasmen der Bauchwandmuskulatur und des Zwerchfells, unkoordinierte Peristalik und Störungen im Zentralnervensystem sind Ursachen der Dysphagie und des gastroösophagealen Refluxes.

Es ist anzustreben, daß geistig behinderte Kinder so früh als möglich röntgenologisch und endoskopisch untersucht werden. Die Fundoplikation sollte erfolgen, bevor Komplikationen auftreten. Besonders Spasmen mit Aspiration und nachfolgender Apnoe sind lebensgefährliche Situationen. Nach der Operation tritt eine wesentliche Besserung in der geistigen und körperlichen Entwicklung ein.

References

Abrahams P, Burkett BFE (1970) Hiatus hernia and gastroesophageal reflux in children and adolescents with cerebral palsy. Aust Pediatr J 6:41

Höllwarth M, Sauer H (1979) Die Entwicklung der Speiseröhrenfunktion bei Neugeborenen – eine manometrische Studie. Z Kinderchir 27:201

Holmes TW (1971) Chalasia, peptic esophagitis and hiatal hernia. A common syndrome in patients with central nervous system disease. Chest 60:441

Johnson DG, Herbst JJ, Oliveros MA, et al (1977) Evaluation of gastroesophageal reflux surgery in children. Pediatrics 59:62

Schärli AF, Rumlova E (1980) Der gastro-ösophageale Reflux im Kindesalter. Helv Chir Acta 47:733

Sondheimer JM, Morris BA (1979) Gastroesophageal reflux among severely retarded children. J Pediatr 94:710

Late Results After Operations for Hiatus Hernia

G. MENARDI[1], G. AUER, and P. EHRLICH

An operation for hiatus hernia in children is not done as often nowadays as it was 10 or 15 years ago. Therefore, it is harder for a pediatric surgical center like Innsbruck, which started in 1968, to amass the patients for a follow-up study that are available in centers which have now existed for four or more decades.

Operative Techniques

Between 1968 and 1981 we operated on 32 children (20 boys and 12 girls) and used various techniques (Table 1) and combinations. In earlier years, Sauer in Innsbruck had preferred hiatopexy, fundoplication, and gastropexy together, a combination which he compared with "trousers being hindered to slide by braces, a belt and a safety pin."

During the last 5 years, we have combined hiatopexy and fundoplication or performed a fundoplication alone.

Age at Operation

The largest number of operations – 11 – were performed in the 1st year of life (Fig. 1); it has to be mentioned that 29 patients were operated upon between 1968 and 1974, and only three since then. Six children suffered from cerebral palsy. Six patients showed a high-grade stenosis of the esophagus and underwent

Table 1. Operations for hiatus hernia 1968–1981 ($n = 32$)

Gastropexy	2
Gastropexy plus fundoplication	3
Hiatopexy	1
Hiatopexy plus gastropexy	5
Hiatopexy plus fundoplication	7
Hiatopexy plus fundoplication plus gastropexy	13
Fundoplication	1

[1]Department of Pediatric Surgery, I. University Clinic of Surgery, Innsbruck, Anichstr. 35, A-6020 Innsbruck/Austria

Progress in Pediatric Surgery, Vol. 18
Ed. by P. Wurnig

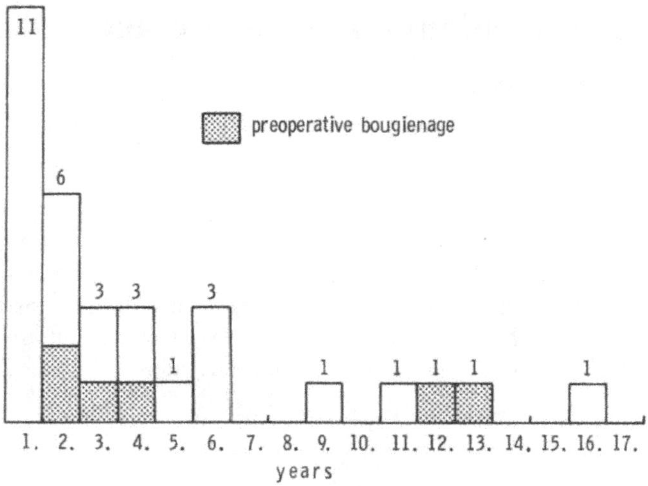

Fig. 1. Age distribution in patients operated upon at the University of Innsbruck between 1968 and 1981 with a diagnosis of hiatus hernia ($n = 32$)

bougienage before the final operation; two had a severe esophagitis, and six had an esophagitis of lesser degree.

Before we discuss the results of the late follow-ups, we have to mention some early complications. We saw one recurrence in a 4-mon-old child 6 weeks after hiatoplexy, fundoplication, and gastropexy; at reoperation, an Allison's hiatopexy was done.

A patient with severe brain damage developed an "upside-down" stomach 4 years after the fundoplication, which itself was intact.

Two children were operated upon in other hospitals for an ileus due to adhesions.

Results

We did late follow-ups in 21 out of 32 operated children. We did not include five children where the parents told us that their children were completely free of any complaints and therefore would not come for a barium study.

We asked our former patient about complaints regarding swallowing, postprandial pains, or bloating; inquired about the ability to belch and to vomit; and asked if the child had undergone any extraction of foreign bodies from the esophagus during the postoperative period. The usual laboratory tests were followed by a barium swallow.

Out of 21 patients (the oldest is 25 years old), three have choking sensations when swallowing larger bites. They all belong to the group of patients who had bougienage before operation because of marked stenosis of the esophagus

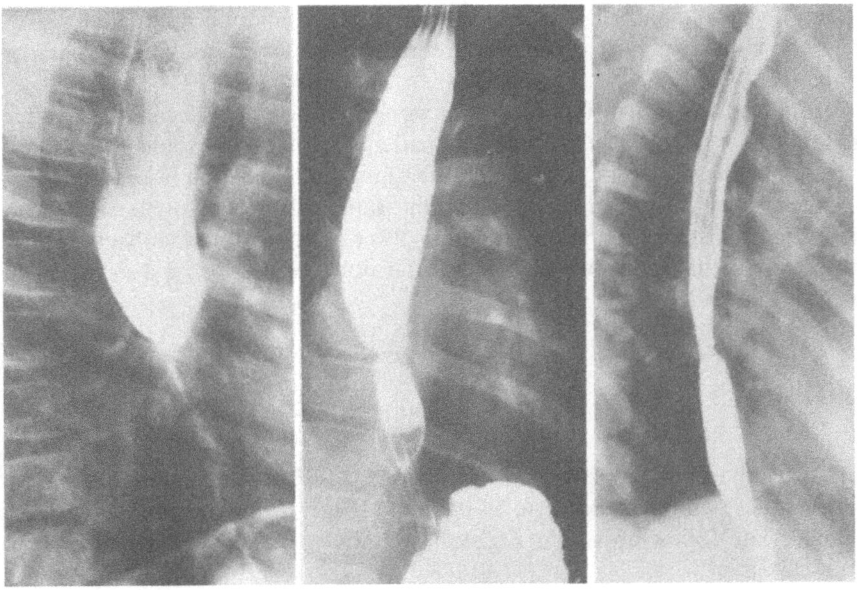

a b c

Fig. 2a–c. Barium passage in a patient who had a hiatopexy plus fundoplication plus gastropexy. **a** Before surgery; **b** 3 years postoperatively, and **c** 8 years postoperatively

Table 2. Late results after operations for hiatus hernia ($n = 21$)

Techniques	Number	Normal radiological findings
Gastropexy	1	1
Gastropexy plus fundoplication	2	2
Hiatopexy	1	1
Hiatopexy plus gastropexy	5	3
Hiatopexy plus fundoplication	3	2
Hiatopexy plus fundoplication plus gastropexy	9	5

(Fig. 2). Two of these patients had to have anesthesia several times to have bits of food removed via endoscope. One of this group had never vomited but did not complain about it. All the others – 20 – were able to belch and to vomit.

There were 18 patients without any complaints, although only 13 patients (including two children with severe preoperative esophagitis) had completely normal barium swallows. Two patients, operated 13 and 14 years ago, had a mild reflux after hiatopexy and gastropexy, but we agree with Rehbein (1979) and call a residual insufficiency of the cardia a good result when the patient is free of complaints.

One 16-year-old patient – 11 years after hiatopexy, fundoplication, and gastropexy – had a massive gastroesophageal reflux without any signs of esophagitis or complaints.

Normal radiological results (Table 2) were due to various techniques: After hiatopexy plus gastropexy we had two patients with gastroesophageal reflux. Stenosis which was present before hiatopexy and fundoplication was still present to a much lesser degree in one patient; the same result was found in the two patients with massive preoperative stenosis after hiatopexy, fundoplication, and gastropexy. In this group we also found the only recurrence of a hernia with massive reflux.

Conclusion

Thirty-two children with gastroesophageal reflux were operated upon using different techniques, which included (in 14 patients) Nissen's fundoplication. Twenty-one had a late follow-up study. Eighteen of these patients were without complaints.

This is in contrast with Schärli's findings (Schärli and Rumlova 1980) of a high morbidity after fundoplication, but we do not agree with Kuffer and Bettex (1974) that a fundoplication is the only right way to surgically correct hiatus hernia in children.

Being familiar with different techniques for correction of hiatus hernia gives us the opportunity to decide from case to case which one to choose.

Summary

Thirty-two children with gastroesophageal reflux were operated by different techniques which included Nissen's fundoplication in 14 patients. Twenty-one patients could be reexamined, eighteen of whom were without complaints. Being familiar with different operative techniques provides the opportunity to decide from case to case which one to choose.

Résumé

32 enfants atteints de reflux gastro-œsophagien ont été opérés selon différentes techniques, y compris la fondoplication selon Nissen dans 14 cas. 21 patients ontpu être réexaminés: 18 ne présentaient plus aucun trouble. Il convient d'être familiarisé avec les différentes techniques opératoires pour décider en toute connaissance de cause de l'opportunité de chacune en fonction de chaque cas bien précis.

Zusammenfassung

32 Kinder mit gastroösophagealem Reflux wurden mit unterschiedlichen Techniken operiert, wobei die Fundoplikation nach Nissen 14mal zur Anwendung kam. 21 Patienten konnten nachuntersucht werden, 18 waren beschwerdefrei. Das Vertrautsein mit verschiedenen Operationstechniken erlaubt die Auswahl der jeweils günstigsten für den Einzelfall.

References

Kuffer F, Bettex M (1974) Die Hiatushernie des Kleinkindes. Z Kinderchir 14(2):153–164

Rehbein F (1979) Kinderchirurgische Operationen. Hippokrates, Stuttgart

Schärli AF, Rumlova E (1980) Der gastro-ösophageale Reflux im Kindesalter. Helv Chir Acta 47:733–747

To Nissen or Not to Nissen

A. F. SCHÄRLI[1]

Nissen's fundoplication has proved to be extremely useful in adults. Because of the simplicity of the procedure and the certain antireflux effect, it is also employed by many pediatric surgeons.

We found the elimination of gastroesophageal reflux and subsequent healing of esophagitis to be sufficient criteria for the use of this technique. A number of unfavorable experiences in recent years, however, have inclined us to call the fundoplication into question: "To Nissen or not to Nissen?"

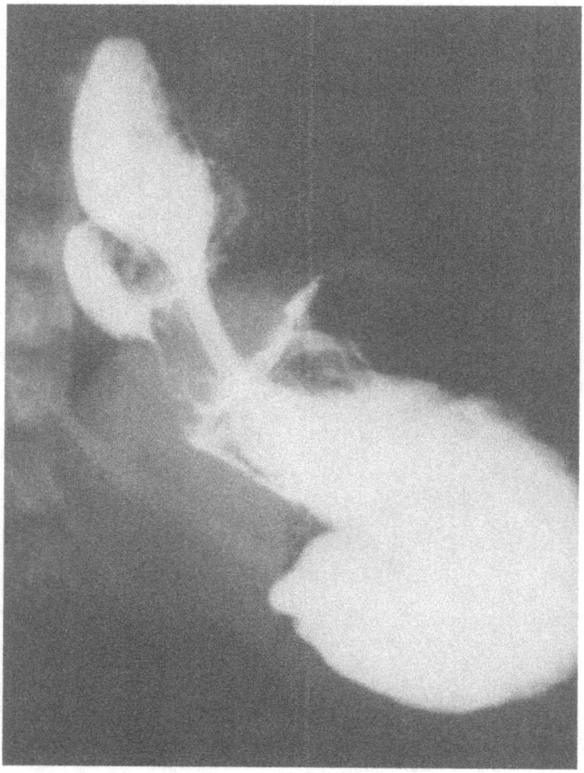

Fig. 1. Parahiatal hernia following Nissen's fundoplication

[1]Department of Pediatric Surgery, Children's Hospital Lucerne, CH-6000 Luzern/Switzerland

Progress in Pediatric Surgery, Vol. 18
Ed. by P. Wurnig

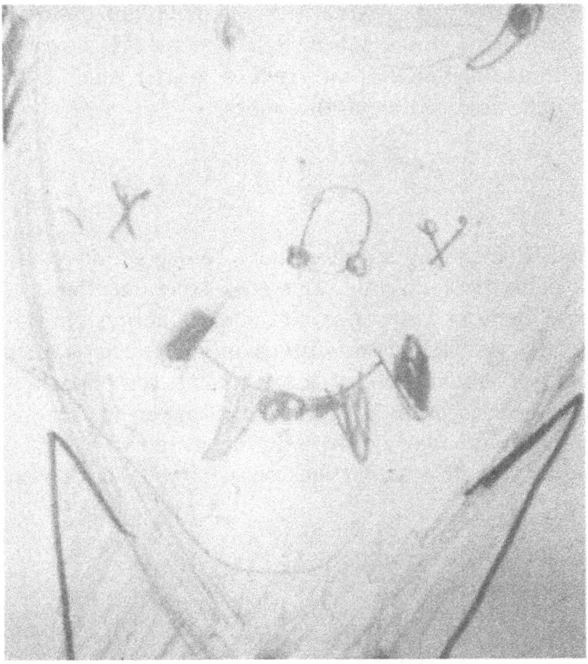

Fig. 2. Neurotic behavior due to bloating syndrome: the patient, who bit his own cheek and lips, draws himself as Dracula

Case Report

Ten years ago, a 3-year-old boy with a history of vomiting and failure to thrive since birth was referred to us with findings typical of gastroesophageal reflux and esophagitis. The vomiting ceased after Nissen's fundoplication was performed; however, severe upper abdominal symtpoms became manifest in the form of a painful sensation of epigastric tension which sometimes increased during meals. Since belching was no longer possible, there was frequent nausea and marked flatulence. Only small meals divided into numerous protions were tolerated.

A contrast study of the esophagus 3 months postoperatively revealed an intact antireflux mechanism, but a parahiatal hernia was also present (Fig. 1).

The surgical reposition of the fundus and narrowing of the hiatus had also failed to alter the clinical picture. The family physician categorized the child as having a neurotic personality.

Eight years following the initial operation, we excised a deep, nomalike ulcer of the left buccal mucosa. Several weeks later, the patient appeared with a deep ulcer of the lower lip. In consultation with a child psychiatrist, a self-portrait came to light in which the patient saw himself as Dracula with bleeding wounds of the check and lower lip (Fig. 2).

The "biting" upper abdominal pains had apparently driven him to bite his own cheek and lip. The behavioral problems thus appeared to have a direct relation to the gas-bloat syndrome. The fundoplication was then reversed, after which both the clinical symptoms and the behavioral problems disappeared.

Discussion

Even in the latest German and English language literature, Nissen's fundoplication is recommended for the pediatric age group. Our own experience has not been encouraging. We attribute our four cases of paraesophageal hernia and two wound dehiscences largely to the marked gastric distension which occurs after Nissen's fundoplication. In addition, about one-half of our patients complained of abdominal bloating. Five children suffered from recurrent upper abdominal cramping. The fundoplication had particularly distressing results in two patients, who subsequently required surgery for obstructive ileus and perforated appendix, respectively (Fig. 3).

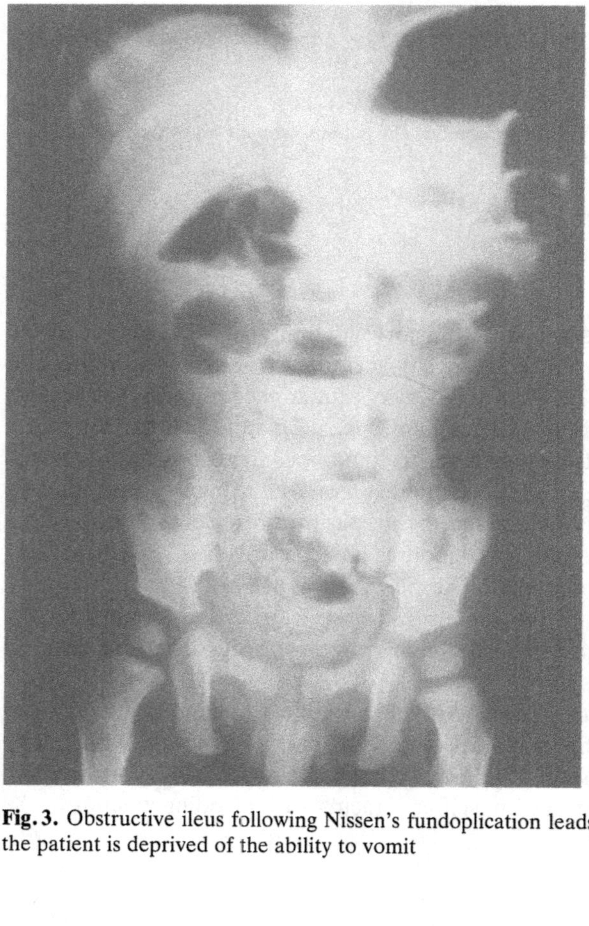

Fig. 3. Obstructive ileus following Nissen's fundoplication leads to severe clinical symptoms, as the patient is deprived of the ability to vomit

In these cases, too, the fundal cuff was restored to its original state.

The bloating syndrome and epigastric cramping do not always diminish postoperatively. In isolated cases, these symptoms have reappeared after an interval of several years.

In a long-term study of 191 cases, Kuffer and Bettex (1974) report on 50 patients (30%) with problems following fundoplication. There were recurrences in 8.4% and 5.6% had developed parahiatal hernias. Two of these patients died of gastric incarceration with perforation.

Since 18% of patients suffer from dysphagia, diarrhea, and bloating, Kuffer writes: "It is advisable to give the child a nasogastric tube as a permanent toilet article."

In the literature, Ashcraft et al. (1978), Ein et al. (1979), DeMeester and Johnson (1976), Henderson (1979), and Herbst et al. (1978) have dealt particularly with the morbidity due to the bloating syndrome.

Conclusions

We are convinced that Nissen's fundoplication is very effective against gastroesophageal reflux. In children, however, the ability to vomit is taken away and the morbidity rate of 25%–50%, depending on author, is very high. Nissen's fundoplication, thus, does not represent the method of choice in children. It is indicated only in cases of short esophagus, for intrathoracic cuff formation, or in patients with cerebral damage for the prevention of active rumination.

A double-row reconstruction of the angle of His in the form of a semi-fundoplication maintains the physiological two-way system of swallowing and eructation, eating, and vomiting.

In answer to the decisive question: To Nissen? – Not to Nissen! –

Summary

Nissen's fundoplication is associated with a high morbidity rate in children. The symptoms are expressed as dysphagia, bloating, diarrhea, and neurotic behavioral changes. On the basis of our own experience, Nissen's fundoplication is not the treatment of choice in children. It is indicated only in cases where a total absence of reflux is tolerable (reflux followed by episodes of apnea, children with cerebral damage, etc.).

Résumé

La fondoplication selon Nissen risque d'entraîner un grand nombre de complications chez l'enfant: dysphagie, ballonements, diarrhées, comportement névrotique. D'après l'auteur, la fondoplication n'est donc pas le procédé de choix chez l'enfant et n'est indiquée que dans les cas exigeant une suppression totale du reflux et rien de moins: cas de reflux suivis d'apnée prolongée, enfants présentant des lésions cérébrales etc.

Zusammenfassung

Die Fundoplikation nach Nissen ist bei Kindern mit einer hohen Komplikationsrate behaftet. Deren Symptome sind Dysphagie, Blähungen, Diarrhöen und neurotische Verhaltensveränderungen. Aufgrund eigener Erfahrungen ist die Fundoplikation nicht als Verfahren der Wahl bei Kindern anzusehen. Sie ist nur bei Fällen indiziert, wo ein völliges Fehlen des Refluxes tolerabel ist (Reflux mit anschließenden Apnoeen, Kinder mit Zerebralschaden etc.).

References

Ashcraft KW, Goodwin CD, Amonry RA, et al (1978) The Thal fundoplication: a simple and safe operative treatment for gastroesophageal reflux. J Pediatr Surg 13:643

De Meester TR, Johnson LF (1976) The evaluation of objective measurements of gastroesophageal reflux and their contribution to patient management. Surg Clin North Am 56:39

Ein SH, Shanding B, Stephens CA, Simpson JS (1979) Partial gastric wrap-around as an alternative procedure in the treatment of hiatal hernia. J Pediatr Surg 14:343

Henderson RD (1979) Nissen hiatal hernia repair: problems of recurrence and continued symptoms. Ann Thorac Surg 28:587

Herbst JJ, Book LS, Bray PF (1978) Gastroesophageal reflux in the "near miss" sudden infant death syndrome. J Pediatr 92:73

Kuffer F, Bettex M (1974) Hiatushernie des Kleinkindes. Früh- und Spätkomplikationen nach Fundoplicatio. Z Kinderchir 14:153

Retroesophageal Hiatal Plasty and Gastropexy in the Treatment of Gastroesophageal Reflux with or Without Hiatus Hernia in Childhood

W. Ch. Hecker[1]

Not every patient with gastroesophageal reflux requires treatment, not to mention surgical treatment. According to the American pediatric surgeon Lucian Leape (1979), closure of the cardia is incomplete in 25%–50% of all infants. Roughly two-thirds of these infants never show symptoms and only one-third become symptomatic. In approximately 75% of the symptomatic infants, symptoms are mild and these children usually undergo treatment by the pediatric practitioner, whereas clinical treatment is necessary in the remaining 25% where most of them, namely 90%, are cured conservatively. Only 10% of this small remaining group require surgery. In about 5% of patients with symptomatic reflux, the symptoms are primarily so severe that immediate pediatric surgical treatment is necessary (Fig. 1).

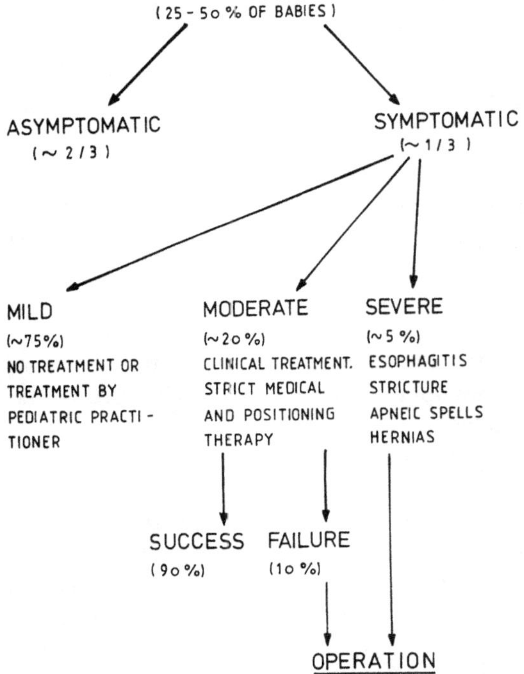

Fig. 1. Forms and therapy in gastroesophageal reflux. (Modified from Leape 1979)

[1]Dept. of Pediatric Surgery of the University Children's Hospital Munich, Lindwurmstr. 4, D-8000 München 2/F.R.G.

Progress in Pediatric Surgery, Vol. 18
Ed. by P. Wurnig

The combination of three diagnostic methods renders the decision for conservative or surgical treatment possible: first, pH monitoring of the esophagus over 24 h shows whether there is a pathologic gastroesophageal reflux or not; second, cineradiography reveals the sort of reflux best classified according to McCanley (1979); third, endoscopy detects inflammatory changes of the esophageal mucosa suitably staged according to Savary-Miller.

We can discriminate between absolute and discussable indications for surgery. Absolute indications are stage II and III esophagitis, according to Savary-Miller, esophageal stricture, Roviralta syndrome, major and eventually medium-sized gastroesophageal refluxes as well as hiatus hernias (except minor forms) in young infants. Among the discussable or relative indications we rank the near miss sudden infant death syndrome, rumination, and recurrent pneumonia. In the last group (pneumonia), an intense diagnostic workup is necessary to reveal how much of it is the responsibility of the gastroesophageal reflux. A scintiscan may be of great help in this situation. Leape (1979) of Boston is convinced that gastroesophageal reflux with subsequent aspiration is the main cause of the sudden infant death syndrome. Before we come to lay down surgical indications, five facts should be considered:

1. An evaluation of the results of conservative treatment in 528 children with hiatus hernia showed that 54% of them were not cured, 19% stopped having symptoms, and 21% were cured (Belohradsky and Hecker 1971).
2. In children with cardial insufficiency with or without hiatus hernia, 19% developed a peptic esophageal stricture, which is difficult to treat (Kuffer and Bettex 1980).
3. Esophagitis is the predecessor of peptic esophageal stenosis.
4. A proven hiatus hernia does not disappear, even if it stops causing symptoms.
5. Fatal cases are observed almost exclusively secondary to complicated and protracted forms.

One can deduce from these facts that pediatric surgeons favor conservative therapy in young infants with minor or eventually medium-sized reflux as well as in minor hiatus hernias. If symptoms do not disappear after 4 weeks of conservative treatment, the operation is indicated.

The aims of surgical treatment of cardial insufficiency with or without hiatus hernia are: to reposition the cardia and the terminal esophagus below the diaphragm, to narrow the diverging diaphragmatic crura, to secure fixation of the cardia and the terminal esophagus below the diaphragm, to reconstruct an acute angle of His, which is important for a reliable prevention of gastroesophageal reflux, and, finally, to tighten the slackened esophagus. This is best achieved by means of the retroesophageal hiatopexy and gastropexy, which was described by Borema and Germes (1955) for adults, adapted for pediatric surgery by Rehbein, and successfully employed by Rehbein (1976), Boix-Ochoa (1979a, b, c), Von Ekesparre (1964), and ourselves. This method provides the reconstruction of physiologic conditions in an ideal manner.

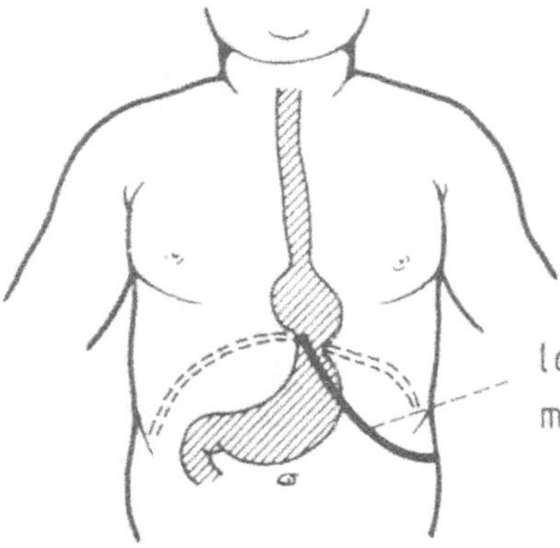

Fig. 2. Operative procedure. Abdominal approach below the left costal margin

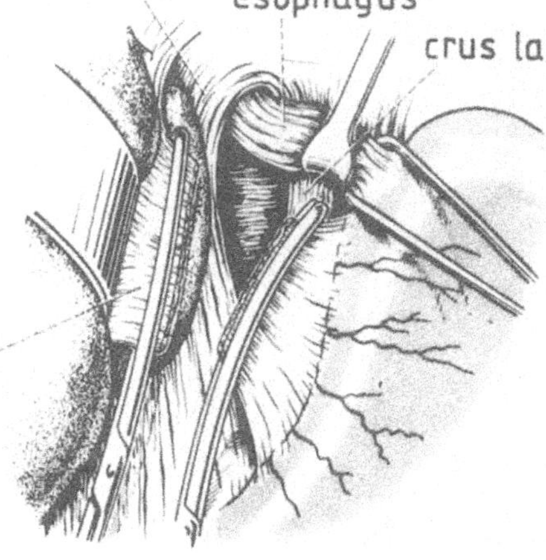

Fig. 3. Operative procedure. Dissection of gastrohepatic omentum; preparation of the hiatus, esophagus, and diaphragmatic crura. Snaring of the esophagus with a rubber catheter

Nissen's fundoplication is also used by many pediatric surgeons (Nissen and Rosetti 1959). This method also prevents the reflux; it establishes, however, an unphysiological anatomical situation, is technically more difficult to perform, and is subject to a higher complication rate. My opinion is that the simpler, more physiologic, and faster method, additionally associated with fewer complications, should be preferred if one can choose between two surgical techniques.

We use the following operative procedure: abdominal approach below the left costal margin (Fig. 2), dissection of the gastrohepatic omentum, preparation of the esophageal hiatus, and preparation and mobilization of the terminal esophagus (Fig. 3). Then we narrow the diverging diaphragmatic crura. To prevent an overcorrection resulting in a stenotic esophageal hiatus, it is useful to have a

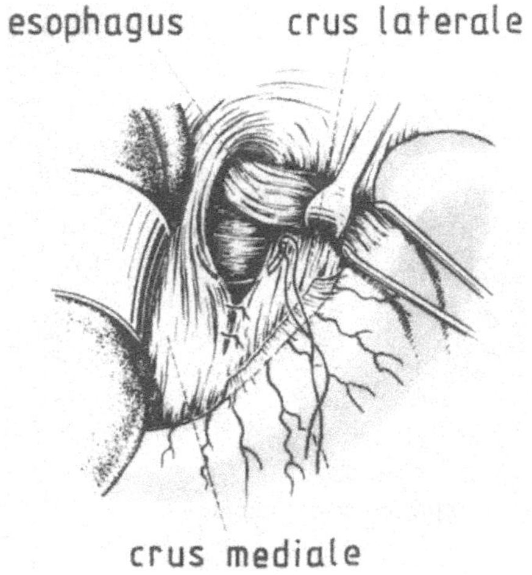

Fig. 4. Operative procedure. The esophagus is held by an angular retractor. Adaptation of the diaphragmatic crura using nonabsorbable sutures, which must not be tied too tightly

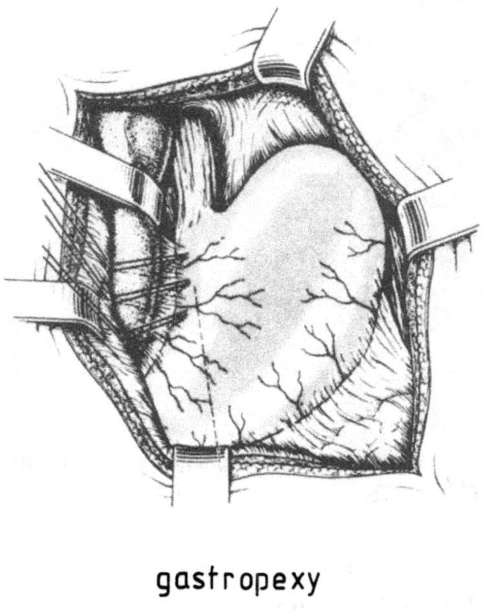

Fig. 5. Operative procedure. Gastropexy is performed by attaching the minor curvature near the cardia to the right anterior abdominal wall using three sutures

thick gastric tube inserted by the anesthetist. For a proper adaptation of the diaphragmatic crura, it is important to grasp a good part of the muscles and to tie them – not too tightly – with nonabsorbable sutures, according to the motto: "Loose though tight enough" (Fig. 4). A good adaptation is achieved if a small dissection swab can be inserted between esophagus and diaphragmatic crura while the gastric tube is in position. Thereafter, a gastropexy is performed, attaching the minor curvature to the right abdominal wall near the cardia by means of nonabsorbable sutures (Fig. 5). Generally the gastric fundus is thus correctly position-

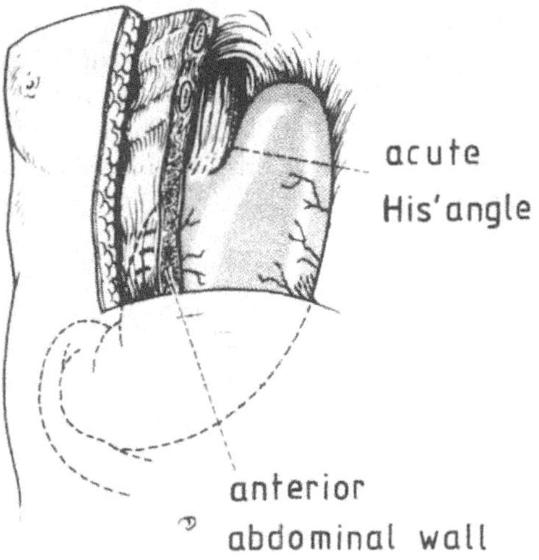

Fig. 6. Operative procedure. The gastropexy exerts moderate traction on the esophagus. The gastric fundus is in the subphrenic space. The acute angle of His provides sufficient closure of the cardia

ed in the subphrenic space, providing an acute angle of His, which is a prior condition for an undisturbed function of the cardia (Fig. 6). If the gastric fundus does not come spontaneously into the desired position, it can be attached to the anterior part of the hiatus with a few sutures.

Cases of esophagitis or esophageal stricture require measures for dilatation later on. For that reason we insert a tie into the esophagus during the operation: Via a small gastrostomy, a nylon suture is attached to the gastric tube and drawn upwards through the nose by the anesthetist. Then the gastrostomy is closed. The distal part of the nylon suture runs through the abdominal wall to the exterior within the region of the gastropexy. This tie serves as a guiding device for repeated esophageal dilatation, starting from the 10th postoperative day.

Since it is our experience that patients with stage II and III esophagitis develop esophageal stenoses following surgery as a consequence of healing, we insert the nylon suture prophylactically in these patients. Dilatation can then be initiated immediately after diagnosis of a beginning stenosis. Control cineradiography is done 3 weeks following surgery. Only esophageal strictures protracted over years cannot be treated by esophageal dilatation. If repeated dilatation over 1½ to 2 years is not successful, the stricture must be corrected surgically. We had to do a resection of the stenosis in two patients and a bypass esophagogastrostomy in five patients. Such operations must always be combined with a pyloroplasty. We try to avoid resection, since this operation is without doubt more time consuming and more complicated than bypass esophagogastrostomy.

Our patient material includes 214 children within 24 years. About one-third of the patients were less than 4 mon old and two-thirds were under 1 year.

Among various forms of cardial insufficiency with or without hiatus hernia, the sliding hernia predominated with 64.9%.

We could follow up 160 patients clinically and radiologically; 83% were without symptoms, and 15% exhibited mild symptoms but were without pathologic radiological findings. These patients suffered occasionally from upper abdominal pain, vomiting, constipation, and sometimes dysphagia. Recurrences occurred in 1.8%, all exclusively following thoracid approaches:

68 of the 214 patients underwent thoracic approaches. From 1963 on, only abdominal approaches were used in the remaining 146 patients. The three cases of recurrence belonged to the 22 thoracic operations which we could follow up, corresponding to a 13% recurrence in this group.

Five patients died, corresponding to a mortality rate of 2.3%. However, no patients have died during the last 12 years. In 1979 Bettex et al. published the results of an inquiry in 1976 including 2789 patiens and reported a mortality rate of 1.47%. I am convinced that we can achieve a mortality rate below 0.5% with the aid of modern intensive care, the right time for surgical intervention, and accurate pretreatment.

Summary

The results of 214 children operated upon for cardial insufficiency with or without hiatus hernia are reported. For follow-up, 160 patients were reexamined: 83% were without symptoms, and 15% showed mild symptoms without pathological radiological findings. Recurrences occurred in 1.8%, all following thoracic operations performed during the early years of this series. A retroesophageal hiatopexy and gastropexy through an abdominal approach was performed on 146 patients. There was no recurrence in this group. Five patients died (2.3%). However, the mortality rate has been zero for the last 12 years.

General aspects, diagnosis, and indication for operation are considered. The operative technique is described in detail.

Résumé

Les auteurs rapportent les résultats de 214 opérations pour insuffisance du cardia avec ou sans hernie chez l'enfant. 160 patients ont été réexaminés 83% d'entre eux ne présentaient plus aucun symptôme. 15% présentaient de discrets symptômes sans que les manifestations radiologiques ne soient pathologiques. Dans 1,8% des cas, il y a eu récidive après intervention par voie thoracique, pendant les premières année de cette étude. 146 patients furent traités par voie abdominale: plastie rétrohiatale et rétro-œsophagienne et gastropexie. Aucune récidive dans ce groupe. 5 patients (2,3%) sont morts. Toutefois aucun décès n'est survenu durant les 12 dernières années.

Les auteurs traitent des aspects généraux, du diganostic et des indications pour les interventions et décrivent en détail la technique opératoire.

Zusammenfassung

Es wird über die Behandlungsergebnisse von 214 operierten Kardiainsuffizienzen mit oder ohne Hiatushernie im Kindesalter berichtet. 160 Patienten konnten nachuntersucht werden, von denen 83% beschwerdefrei waren; 15% wiesen geringe Beschwerden auf, jedoch ohne pathologischen Röntgenbefund. Bei 1,8% der Fälle kam es zum Rezidiv, das ausschließlich nach der früher verwendeten thorakalen Operation auftrat. 146 Patienten wurden abdominell mit der retroösophagealen Hiatusplastik und Gastropexie behandelt. Hier zeigte sich kein Rezidiv. 5 Patienten (2,3%) starben. In den letzten 12 Jahren wurde kein letaler Ausgang mehr beobachtet.

Allgemeine Gesichtspunkte, Diagnose und Operationsindikation werden dargestellt. Die Operationstechnik wird detailliert beschrieben.

References

Belohradsky BH, Hecker WC (1971) Problematik und Klinik der Cardiainsuffizienz mit und ohne Hiatushernie. Ergeb Chir Orthopäd 55:123

Bettex M, Oesch-Amrein J, Kuffer F (1979) Mortality after operation for hiatus hernia. Progr Ped Surg 13:245–252. Urban & Schwarzenberg, Munich Baltimore

Boix-Ochoa J (1979a) Pressure studies in GER/hiatal hernia. In: Gastroesophageal reflux. Ross Laboratories, Columbos, Ohio

Boix-Ochoa J (1979b) GI pressure studies in GER/hiatal hernia. In: Gastroesophageal reflux. Ross Laboratories, Columbus, Ohio

Boix-Ochoa J (1979c) pH monitoring in GER/hiatal hernia. In: Gastroesophageal reflux. Ross Laboratories, Columbus, Ohio

Borema J, Germes R (1955) Fixation of the lesser curvature of the stomach to the anterior abdominal wall after reposition of the hernia through the oesophageal hiatus. Arch Chir Neurol 7:351

Ekesparre W von (1964) Operatives Vorgehen bei der kindlichen Hiatushernie. Langenbeck's Arch Klin Chir 308:133

Kuffer F, Bettex M (1980) Hiatushernie und gastro-oesophagealer Reflux. Padiatr Praxis Klinik 2:1366

Leape LL (1979) Gastroeosophageal reflux as a cause of the sudden infant death syndrome. In: Gastroesophageal reflux. Ross Laboratories, Columbus, Ohio

McCanley RG (1979) Radiological demonstration of gastroesophageal reflux and hiatal hernia in infants and children. In: Gastroesophageal reflux. Ross Laboratories, Columbus, Ohio

Nissen R, Rosetti M (1959) Die Behandlung der Hiatushernie und Refluxoesophagitis mit Gastropexie und Fundoplikation. Georg Thieme, Stuttgart

Rehbein F (1976) Kinderchirurgische Operationen. Hippokrates, Stuttgart

Small Bowel Esophagoplasty with Vascular Microanastomoses in the Neck for Treatment of Esophageal Burns in Childhood

J. Prévot, M. Lepelley, and M. Schmitt[1]

Introduction

Esophageal burns and peptic esophagitis, though well known for a long time, have become more and more important in our practice during the last 10 years. This fact is highly correlated with the increasingly routine use of extremely aggressive household cleaning agents, which are also packed in very attractive containers. Moreover, this fact depends also on the larger geographic area which we cover, including not only the Lorraine region but also some French-speaking African countries. For these reasons, we have had to treat 25 children with esophageal burns and one with peptic esophagitis during the last 15 years in whom dilatation would have been entirely inadequate.

Since it is impossible to nourish the children via gastrostomy throughout their life, one has to resort to esophagus-replacing operations. In the majority of the cases (23 out of 26), we could realize esophagoplasties by interposition of the isoperistaltic transverse colon with a pedicle containing the left colic artery, according to the technique of Belsey. This technique provides the advantage of a wide and useful bowel segment which is relatively resistant to the gastric juice. Moreover, it is not particularly disfiguring to the children, since the whole procedure is performed via thoracotomy in the left 7th intercostal space, except for the esophagocolonic anastomosis in the neck. This procedure requires, however, some technical finesse in order to establish a straight tube without kinking, particularly at the level of the diaphragm. We have repeatedly described the particulars in the French literature. One out of 23 children who had a colonic interposition died of purulent mediastinitis. Two children had to undergo reoperation for correction of kinking above the diaphragm. Reintervention in the neck had to be done in seven children for correction of fistulas or anastomotic stenosis.

If the colon cannot be used – a situation which is rather rare –, esophagus substitution can be achieved by means of Gavriliu's technique, using the major curvature of the stomach. We do not favor this method, since on the one hand the stomach itself may not be entirely intact, and on the other hand the tube thus constructed may be too narrow and the gastric mucosa may itself cause problems for the cervical esophagus with which it will be in contact, i.e., esophagitis.

We could not use the classic operation in two recent cases and solved the problem by use of a small bowel graft in which the vessels were carefully prepared

[1] Children's Hospital Nancy, Allée du Morvan, F-54511 Vandœuvre les Nancy Cedex/France

Progress in Pediatric Surgery, Vol. 18
Ed. by P. Wurnig

and anastomosed in the cervical region. We want to present these two cases, the technique applied, and the results in detail.

Case 1

Sebastian A., born 6 January 1971. The boy suffered from severe ulcerative colitis from his 3rd year on which was treated conservatively; however, colectomy was repeatedly discussed. When he became 5 years old in January 1976, he swallowed a large dose of Destop, a powerful household drain cleaner. Soon he developed severe esophageal stricture, which was resistant to both medical treatment and dilatation. A gastrostomy was established and esophagus replacement became necessary (Fig. 1). The colon was unserviceable due to edema, fibrous thickening, and hemorrhagic changes (Fig. 2). Esophagoplasty was performed in January 1977, according to the method of Gavriliu, using the stomach. Immediately postoperatively, the result seemed to be satisfactory, but then progressively, the boy developed extensive stenosis which included the upper half of the gastric tube. Progression continued despite numerous dilatations and a revision of the upper anastomosis (Fig. 3). A new gastrostomy had to be established. Several episodes of intestinal hemorrhaging showed the persistence and the severity of the ulcerative colitis.

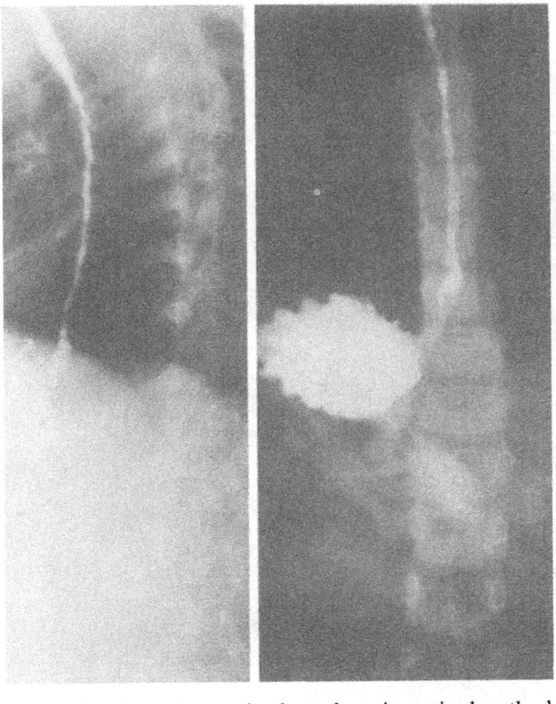

Fig. 1. Esophageal stenosis, throughout its entire length, due to ingestion of a caustic liquid

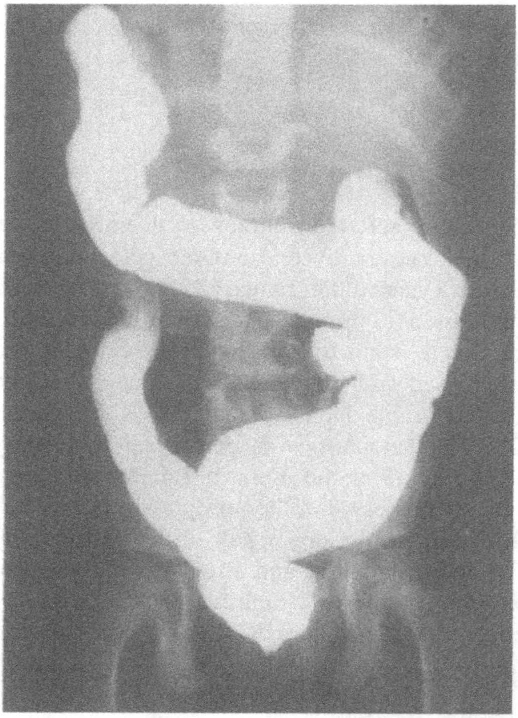

Fig. 2. Typical picture of ulcerative colitis: Disappearance of haustra, with a rigid, atrophic colon

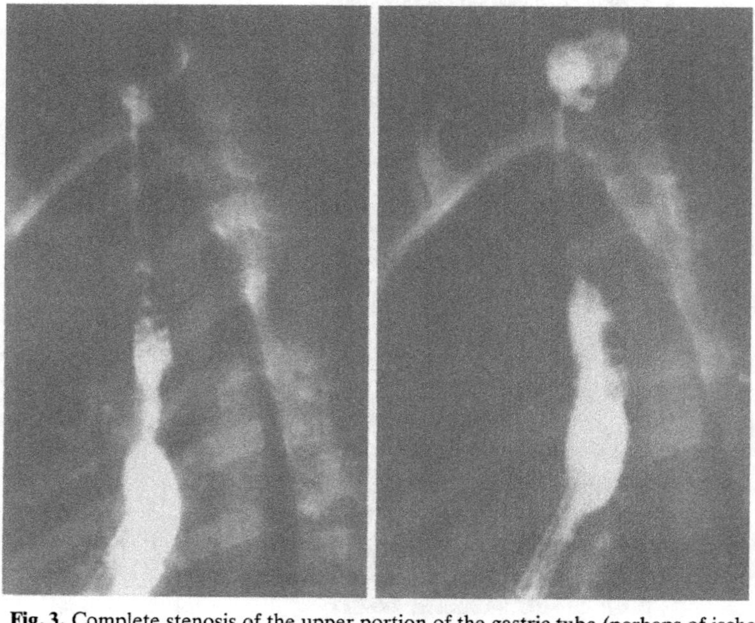

Fig. 3. Complete stenosis of the upper portion of the gastric tube (perhaps of ischemic origin)

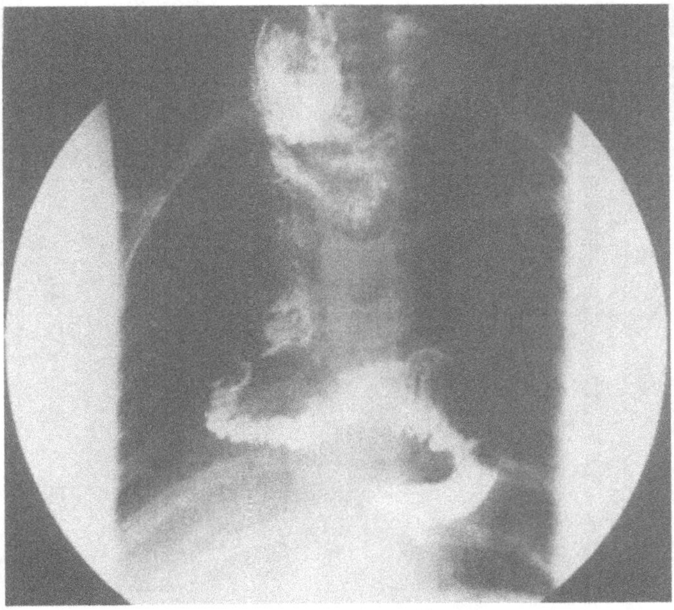

Fig. 4. Opacification of the thoracic portion of the graft

We decided to transplant a segment of small bowel which was done on 10 December 1979, under the direction of Dr. Germain, an assistant of Prof. Roux of Paris. The postoperative course was uncomplicated: Oral nutrition was started on the 10th postoperative day; from the 3rd week on the boy was nourished exclusively orally. Gastrostomy was withdrawn 2 mon later. Swallowing is normal, except for mild disturbances if the boy drinks a large amount of fluid too quickly (Figs. 4 and 5).

Results of the last follow-up show that he eats normally, he is of normal weight and height for his age, and his ulcerative colitis is perfectly stable (Fig. 6).

Case 2

Adil G., a Moroccan boy with a slight encephalopathy, swallowed a large amount of potash (potassium hydroxide) in April 1979 at the age of 6. Immediately, a gastrostomy was established and repeated dilatations were performed. The esophageal stricture became quicked impassable, even for minute amounts of liquid. This led to numerous pulmonary complications. The boy was in poor general condition when we performed colonic interposition, according to Belsey, on 18 November 1981. During the laparotomy, we saw marked fibrosis of the stomach, complicated by an ulcer of the posterior wall, and multiple lesions caused by the burn. The vessel supply to the colon was unfavorable and there was

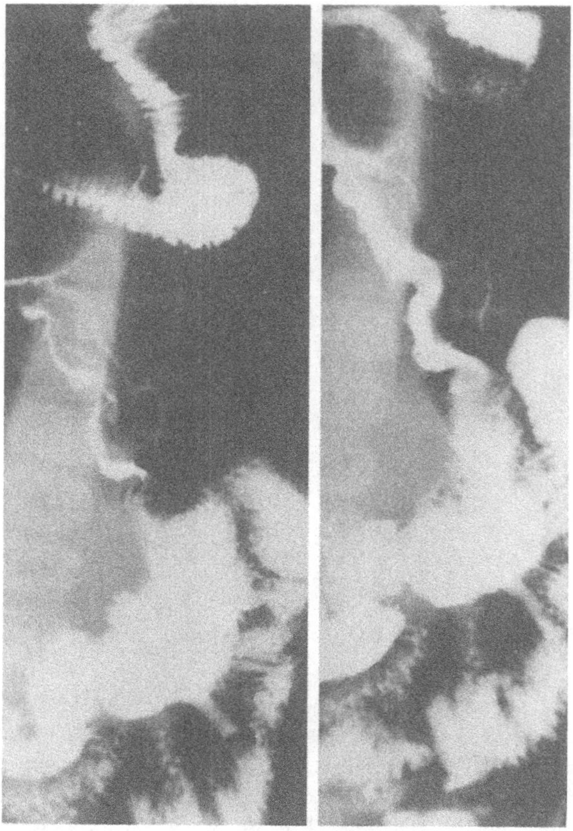

Fig. 5. Satisfactory transit despite the undulations

significant edema of the transverse mesocolon. However, the operation seemed to provide a satisfactory result and the postoperative course was uneventful for 10 days. From then on acute febrile complications appeared, due to a large perforation of the graft. Immediate surgical reintervention was necessary and revealed subtotal necrosis of the graft. The boy, still bearing the gastrostomy, finally recovered.

Since the stomach could not be used due to its severe fibrosis, we performed a small bowel transplantation 8 mon later in June 1982. Postoperative course was uneventful. Restarting oral nutrition, however, was difficult for psychologic reasons. Anastomotic stenosis required surgical revision in the neck in September 1982. Since then, oral nutrition has been normal, except for some difficulty when ingestion is rapid (like in the previous patient). The boy is in good general condition.

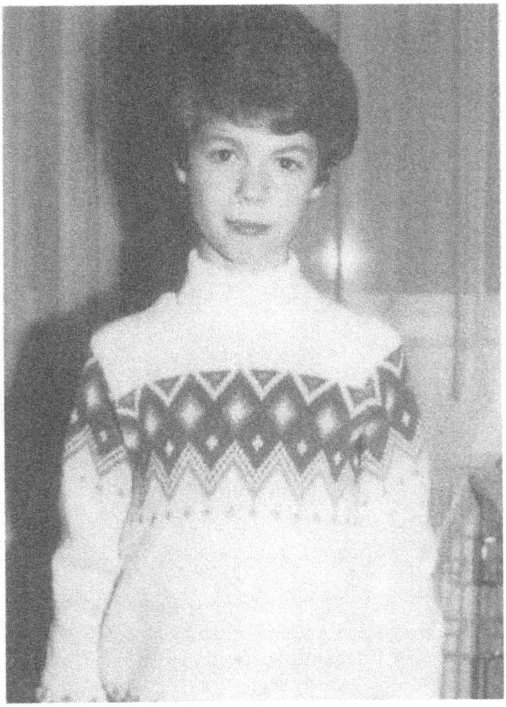

Fig. 6. Our patient, 4 years after his transplant, at 12 years of age (no. 2)

Discussion

Technical Considerations

The choice of which portion of intestine to use almost always depends on local conditions. In our first patient, there was a good vessel supply of the jejunum; in the second patient, we used the distal ileum. In each case, vessel preparation must be done as near as possible to the root of the superior mesenteric vessels to obtain the largest possible vessel calibers. The intestine, when cooled to between 10° and 15°C, was affected. It is advantageous to do the bowel resection and anastomosis, create a wide retrosternal channel, and prepare the cervical vessels *before* the resection of the blood vessels feeding the graft. Once this is done, the bowel is immediately brought into retrosternal position and the vessels are anastomosed (Fig. 7). As far as arterial blood supply is concerned, any readily accessible branch of the external carotid may be used. In the first patient, we indeed used the inverted trunk of the external carotid artery (Fig. 8); in the second case, we had to place the anastomosis very low in order to obtain an end-to-side anastomosis between the bowel artery and the trunk of the common carotid artery. For the venous side, one must always use the internal jugular, paying attention to providing a lie which

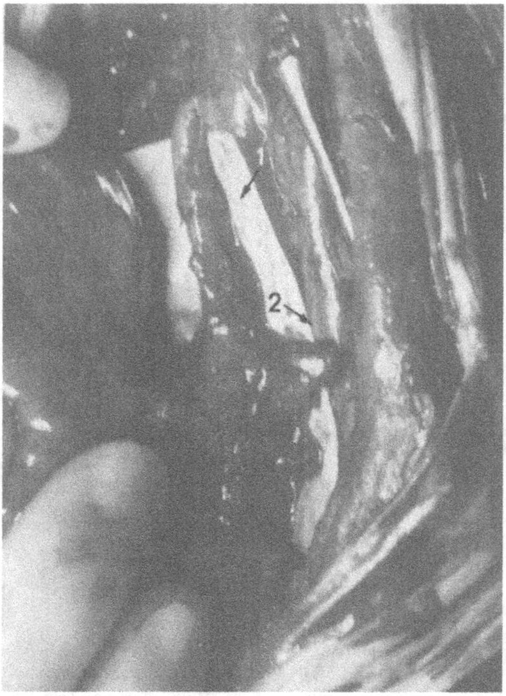

Fig. 7. Operative view of the arterial anastomosis *(arrow 1)* and the venous anastomosis *(arrow 2)*, which is less easily seen

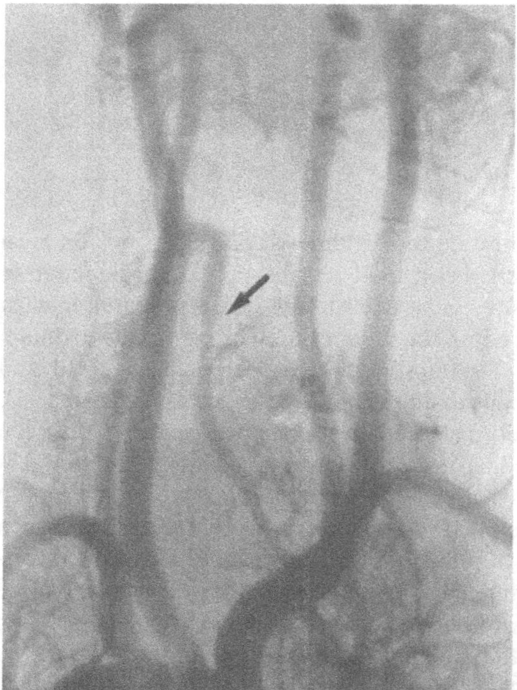

Fig. 8. Follow-up arteriography done 1 year postoperatively. One can clearly see the trunk of the external carotid artery turned downward and the anastomosis with the intestinal artery

provides an unimpaired blood flow. Naturally, a microscope must be used. After the blood vessels are attached, the two ends of the small intestine graft can be anastomosed to the cervical esophagus and to the posterior wall of the stomach. Anticoagulation is not necessary.

Functional Considerations

There seem to be several barriers standing in the way of the use of small bowel as an esophageal substitute, as far as function is concerned. The first is the small caliber of the small intestine and its slow peristalsis, quite different from that of the esophagus. These disproportions seem not to be important in practice, since the digestive tract adapts well to rapid contractions, additionally favored by the upright position of the patient. It is only the attempt at swallowing a large mass that is overwhelming for the graft. The children, however, are aware of this fact and become familiar with the new situation very quickly.

The small bowel graft always looks very bent, since it cannot be fully straightened without severely impairing the blood supply. Experience shows, however, that transit is quick and completely unaffected by the impressive bends.

Finally, we could not observe any problems, even transitory ones, resulting from contact between gastric juice and the graft. The lower anastomosis, however, is always established in such a way as to prevent reflux by attaching the bowel graft to the posterior wall of the stomach.

Conclusions

Nowadays microsurgery allows the difficulties of vascular microanastomoses to be easily overcome. Therefore one could be tempted to regard the ileal graft as an ideal esophageal substitute if the latter is damaged. We do not believe in this absolutely for various reasons:

1. Although the graft usually adapts well to the new situation, its caliber may prove to be too narrow for larger pieces of food.
2. Microanastomoses of vessels always tend to thrombose.
3. But perhaps the most important problem is that because of its sinuosity, nearly 1 m of small bowel is necessary to span the distance between neck and stomach, meaning a more important functional loss as compared with esophageal replacement using the colon.

Nevertheless, esophageal replacement by small bowel transplantation, using a pedicule in the neck, is a very good method of esophageal substitution, and there is no doubt that its use will be increasingly indicated in children.

Summary

Replacement of the esophagus may become mandatory in esophageal burns if dilatation treatment is unsuccessful. Normally, the isoperistaltic transverse colon placed in the neck is used for this purpose. The use of the major curvature of the stomach, according to Gavriliu, may also be considered. In two of our patients, these techniques could not be applied, and we transplanted a portion of the small bowel into the neck, with the blood supply to the pedicule being provided by vascular microanastomosis in the cervical region. The functional results were very satisfying in both cases, despite of the bent appearance of the grafts. At long-term follow-up, there have been no major, particularly peptic, complications. The two cases and the technique applied are described.

Résumé

Dans les œsophagites caustiques, le remplacement de l'œsophage peut s'imposer lorsque le traitement par dilatations est inefficace ou dépassé. Habituellement les auteurs utilisent dans ce but le colon transverse monté au cou en situation isopéristaltique. L'utilisation de la grande courbure gastrique peut aussi être envisagée selon le procédé de Graviliu.

Dans deux cas, le recours à ces deux techniques s'étant révélé impossible, les auteurs ont transplanté au cou une anse grêle dont le pédicule a été anastomosé aux vaisseaux du cou par microsutures vasculaires. Le résultat fonctionnel a été très satisfaisant dans les deux cas malgré l'aspect très tortueux de la plastie œsophagienne. A distance, il n'y a pas eu de complication particulière peptique notamment.

La technique et les modalités d'anastomose sont détaillées après la description des cas.

Zusammenfassung

Bei Ösophagusverätzungen kann der Ersatz der Speiseröhre zwingend notwendig sein, wenn die Behandlung durch Bougierung unwirksam ist. Gewöhnlich wird dazu das Colon transversum benutzt, das unter isoperistalischen Verhältnissen zum Hals hochgezogen wird. Die Verwendung der großen Magenkurvatur nach Gavriliu kann ebenfalls in Betracht gezogen werden. Bei 2 Fällen waren diese Techniken nicht anwendbar, und die Autoren transplantierten eine Dünndarmschlinge, deren Gefäße im Halsgebiet mit den Halsgefäßen in Mikrotechnik anastomosiert wurden. Das funktionelle Resultat war trotz des sehr gewundenen Aussehens der Ösophagoplastik in beiden Fällen sehr zufriedenstellend. Es traten keine besonderen, insbesondere keine peptischen Komplikationen auf. Technik und Problematik werden nach den Fallbeschreibungen erläutert.

References

Germain M, Patricio J, Gremillet C, Delavierre P, Dehoux P, Voudron J, Loisance DY (1977) Oesophagoplastie totale par anse jéjunale avec micro-anastomoses vasculaires au cou. Etude expérimentale. Chirurgie 103:264–267

Green GE, Som ML (1966) Free grafting and revascularisation of intestine. Replacement of the cervical esophagus. Sugery 60:1012–1017

Kasai M, Abo S, Makino K, Yoshiba S, Taguchi Y (1965) Reconstruction of the cervical esophagus with a pedicled jejunal graft. Surg Gynecol Obstet 121:102–106

Longmire W (1947) A modification of the Roux's technique for antethoracicoesophageal reconstruction. Anastomosis of the mesenteric and internal mammary blood vessels. Surgery 22:94–100

Noirclerc M, Malmejac C, Paoli JM, Dor J (1967) Oesophagoplastie par transplantation intestinale au cou. Etude expérimentale et clinique. Ann Chir Thorac Cardiovasc 6:154–159

Peters CR, McKee DM, Berry BE (1971) Pharyngoesophageal reconstruction with revascularized jejunal transplants. Am J Surg 121:675–678

Rudler JC, Lafargue P (1953) Les oesophagoplasties avec le tube digestif. 55ème Congrès de Chirurgie. Paris. Presses Universitaires de France, pp 19–136

Vayre P, Germain M, Jost JL, Hureau J, Roux M (1980) Oesophagoplastie pour cancer de l'oesophage par transplant d'une anse grêle isopéristaltique en Y au cou par voie souscutanée avec micro-anastomoses vasculaires. Ann Chir 34(6):396–399

Vergnolle M, Videau J (1977) Etude expérimentale des oesophagoplasties préthoraciques jéjunales avec réimplantation vasculaire au cou chez le chien. Bordeaux Méd 10:57

Yudin S (1944) Oesophagoplastie préthoracique. Surg Gynecol Obstet 78:561–585

Follow-up Examinations of Conservatively and Surgically Treated Children with Hiatus Hernia

U. A. Bernhard and D. H. Shmerling[1]

Introduction

The symptoms and the clinical picture of esophageal hiatus hernia depend largely on the presence and degree of gastroesophageal reflux. It is reflux which produces the severe complications, such as esophagitis, secondary scar contracture, aspiration, and bronchopneumonia. The main purpose of therapy is directed toward the prevention of such complications.

In this investigation the clinical characteristics, the treatment, and the results in 65 patients with hiatus hernia and gastroesophageal reflux are described.

Patients and Methods

The 65 patients with hiatus hernia proved by radiological investigations admitted between January 1966 and December 1976 to the University Children's Hospital

Table 1. Number of patients and type of treatment over the 1st week, according to radiological findings

Type of hernia	Treatment		Total
	Surgical	Conservative	
Forme mineure			
Type 1: Chalasia of the cardia			
a. with slight reflux	1	8	9
b. with massive reflux	1	10	11
Type 2: Sliding hiatus hernia with small pouch	11	23	34
Forme majeure			
Type 3: Sliding hiatus hernia with large pouch	6	4	10
Type 4: Sliding hiatus hernia combined with paraesophageal hernia	1	–	1
Total	20	45	65

[1]Dept. of Gastroenterology, University Children's Hospital, Steinwiesstr. 75, CH-8032 Zürich/ Switzerland

Progress in Pediatric Surgery, Vol. 18
Ed. by P. Wurnig

Zürich were examined. The diagnosis was made by barium swallow and the radiological discovery of a hiatus hernia with reflux classified according to Sauvegrain (1957) into *forme mineure* and *forme majeure* (Table 1).

All the important factors were extracted from the case sheets, including the past history, the radiological diagnosis, and the therapy.

In spring 1978 (14 mon to 10 years after first admission to hospital), a questionnaire was sent to the parents of the children, inquiring after the type of treatment the child received at home, the duration of the symptoms, and whether any symptoms were still observed.

Of the 65 parents who received the questionnaire, 39 responded. If the parents replied positively to the questions: "Were there still complaints after hospitalization or after treatment had been discontinued," the children were asked to come in for a follow-up examination. This comprised the taking of a detailed clinical history, clinical examination, and estimation of the hemoglobin concentration. If there were the necessary indications, an esophagoscopy was performed.

Results

Hospitalization

Age at Diagnosis

The majority of the 65 patients (67.7%) were less than 6 mon old when admitted to hospital; 81.6% were less than 1 year old. The four children (6.1%) who were older than 10 years had severe changes. There was one patient with a vague dysmorphic syndrome, one with the Prader-Willi-Labhart syndrome, and two with infantile paralysis.

Symptoms

The most frequent symptoms were vomiting, failure to gain weight, and infections of the upper respiratory tract.

In 64 patients (99%), vomiting occurred. In the majority it started during the 1st week of life and was either projectile or simple regurgitation of stomach contents. Hematemesis occurred in 30 patients. In 35 patients, the vomitus was benzidine-positive.

On admission to hospital the weight was under the 3rd percentile in 41.5% of the patients (measured according to the Boston percentile table). In 21 or 32.3% of the patients, the weight was between the 3rd and the 10th percentile. The exact distribution can be seen from Fig. 1.

Recurrent infections of the upper respiratory tract had been observed in 12 patients.

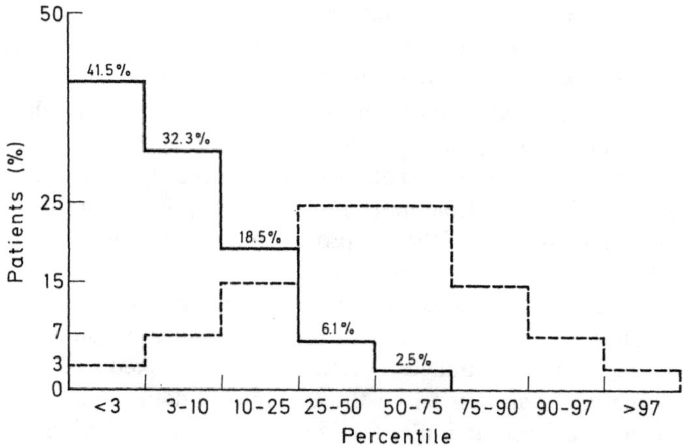

Fig. 1. Weight of the patients on admission to hospital. ——— Patients, —·—·—· normal children

Laboratory Investigations

In half the patients, either the feces or the vomitus was benzidine-positive.

There were 19 patients who suffered from anemia, with a hemoglobin concentration of 11 g% or lower. There was no relationship between the degree of anemia and the severity of the hiatus hernia.

Radiological Findings

Aspiration pneumonia was diagnosed radiologically in six patients.

The hernias found on esophagogram carried out at the first admission to hospital were classified as *forme mineure* and *forme majeure* (Table 1).

Of the 34 patients with an *forme mineure,* the primary treatment was conservative in 23 cases. In six patients (two children with chalasia of the cardia type 1b and four children of type 2), conservative treatment was not successful and surgery had to be carried out later on. In two patients with chalasia of the cardia, there was such a severe reflux esophagitis and massive reflux or secondary scar stenosis of the esophagus that primary operations were carried out.

In 11 patients, esophagitis could be diagnosed either by radiology or endoscopy. One patient already has a secondary stenosis at the gastroesophageal junction on admission.

Additional Findings

In 16 patients, additional clinical findings were seen. Four children suffered from cerebral paralysis, three from the Roviralta syndrome, and a further three had been operated upon for left-sided diaphragmatic eventration. Other findings occurred only singly and appeared to be accidental combinations.

Treatment

In 20 patients, a primary operation was carried out. In six further patients, who were initially unsuccessfully treated conservatively, a fundoplication had to be performed as a secondary step. The distribution of the types of operation carried out can be seen from Table 2.

In 45 children (69.2%), conservative therapy was carried out which was unsuccessful in six, necessitating operation on second admission to hospital. Table 3 shows the number of children treated conservatively according to the radiological type.

Table 2. Type of operation carried out classified according to the original radiological finding. Four patients (a, b, c, d) had to undergo more than one operation

Hiatus hernia	Operation	Number
Type 1a	Fundoplication (severe esophagitis)	1 (a)
1b	Fundoplication (esophageal stenosis)	1 (b)
	Fundoplication after unsuccessful conservative treatment	2
Type 2	Fundoplication	10 (c, d)
	Fundoplication after unsuccessful conservative treatment	4
	Esophagogastropexy	1
Type 3	Fundoplication	3
	Fundoplication/gastropexy	1
	Esophagogastropexy	1
	Fundoplication/gastrostomy	1
Type 4	Fundoplication	1

Table 3. Number of children treated conservatively classified according to the original radiological finding

Hiatus hernia	Number of patients with similar radiological findings	Number of patients treated conservatively during hospitalization
Type 1a	9	8 (88.8%)
Type 1b	11	10 (90.9%)[a]
Type 2	34	23 (67.6%)[b]
Type 3	10	4 (40.0%)
Type 4	1	0

[a] Two of the 10 later had operative treatment
[b] Four of the 23 later had operative treatment

The conservative therapy consisted mainly of three measures: sitting the patient up (100%), thickening of the feed (68.8%), and antacids (57.7%). If necessary, this treatment was combined with iron therapy (44.4%) and/or sedatives (28.8%).

(The percentage in brackets indicates how often the treatment had to be carried out.)

Questionnaire

Of the 65 questionnaires sent out, 39 were returned. The type of treatment related to the radiological findings as shown in Table 4.

One patient with a Prader-Willi-Labhart syndrome was treated conservatively, was radiologically type 3, and died 2 years after hospitalization. This patient is not included in the following analysis.

Table 4. Type of treatment in relation to the radiological findings abstracted from the questionnaires

Hiatus hernia	Treatment	
	Surgical	Conservative
Type 1a	1	5
1b	3	3
Type 2	8	12
Type 3	5	1
Type 4	1	0

Table 5. Type and frequency of home therapy

Type of treatment	Treatment	
	Conservative ($n = 16$)	Surgical ($n = 7$)
Head elevated	16	3
Thickened feed	8	1
Antacids	5	5
Iron therapy	4	4
Sedatives	4	1

Therapy at Home

In 41.1% of the surgically treated patients and in 76.1% of the conservatively treated patients (total 23), treatment had been prescribed after discharge from hospital and had been carried out. Parents of 15 patients stated that they had not carried out any treatment after discharge from hospital, although in seven of these patients, treatment had been prescribed.

The type of treatment, according to the parents, can be seen from Table 5.

Duration of Therapy

The duration of therapy varied markedly. If therapy was necessary after discharge from hospital, it lasted more than 1 year in 45% of the surgically treated patients and in 30% of the conservatively treated patients.

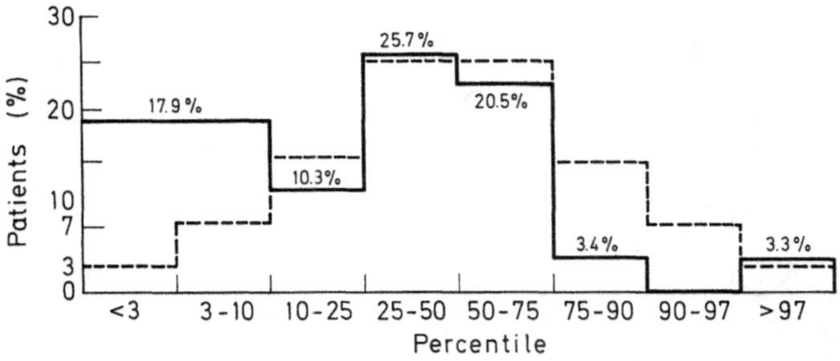

Fig. 2. Distribution of weight according to the replies received to the questionnaire. ——— Patients, —·—·—· normal children

Distribution of Body Weight

According to the answers received to the questionnaires, seven children (17.9%) had a weight under the 3rd percentile; three of these children suffered from cerebral paralysis and one is still under treatment. Figure 2 shows the exact distribution of weight.

Patients Free from Symptoms

In 26 of the total of 38 patients (68.4%), the parents stated that after cessation of therapy or after the last hospitalization respectively, they were free from symptoms. The distribution according to the type of hiatus hernia and the treatment received can be seen from Table 6.

It is noticeable that all children with hiatus hernia type 1a are symptom free. Unfortunately it is impossible to make any definite statement about the results of conservative treatment in patients with hiatus hernia type 3. The only parents who answered the questionnaire were those whose child had a Prader-Willi-Labhart syndrome and had died. The cause of death could not be ascertained.

Table 6. Number of patients without symptoms classified according to the original radiological findings and the treatment received. The percentages relate to the number of questionnaires returned (see Table 4)

Hiatus hernia	Treatment	
	Surgical	Conservative
Type 1a	1 (100.0%)	5 (100.0%)
1b	2 (66.6%)	2 (66.6%)
Type 2	5 (62.5%)	7 (58.3%)
Type 3	3 (60.0%)	0
Type 4	1 (100.0%)	0

Table 7. Follow-up examination findings in patients who continued to have complaints

Patient, date of birth	Findings/therapy		Questionnaire	Follow-up examination
S.D. 30 Jul 1965	Nov 1965 Jan 1968	*Forme mineure,* type 2: conservative therapy *Forme mineure,* type 2: conservative therapy	Vomiting	Vomiting after exertion at night. Retrosternal feeling of pressure. X-ray: *forme mineure,* type 2, without esophagitis Hb: 12.9 g% Weight: 3rd percentile Height: 3rd to 10th percentile
B.R. 19 Nov 1960	Perinatal cerebral hemorrhage: spastic tetraplegia May 1964 Jun 1966	 *Forme mineure:* conservative therapy *Forme mineure* with reflux esophagitis and anemia (Hb 8.7 g%): conservative therapy	Vomiting Constipation	1972–1974 practically no vomiting; since 1974 occasional vomiting at night Hb: 15.3 g% Weight: 3rd percentile Height: 3rd percentile
H.R. 16 Mar 1965	May 1965 Sep 1965 Jan 1968 Oct 1972 Nov 1973 Apr 1975	*Forme mineure,* type 2: eventration of diaphragm and fundoplication Esophageal stenosis; anemia; dilatation with bougies Severe psychomotor retardation with microcephaly and dystrophy Esophageal stenosis with reflux esophagitis Fundoplication (diaphragmatic plication) Vagotomy; pyloroplasty Esophagoscopy: slight stenosis and shallow ulcus distally Esophagoscopy: no pathology	Vomiting Difficulties in swallowing	Retrograde burning pain when coughing and bending down; rarely feeling of pressure retrosternally Hb: 11.4 g% Weight: 3rd percentile Height: 3rd to 10th percentile

A.F. 20 Feb 1966		Jejunal atresia. Side-to-side anastomosis	Difficulties in swallowing and heartburn	Difficulties in swallowing, especially solid food; retrosternal pain when lying down
	Jul 1966	Cardial insufficiency with reflux esophagitis and stenosis of esophagus Aspiration pneumonia Fundoplication; bougienage		
	Oct 1967	Esophageal stenosis Esophagogastropexy; bougienage Gastrostomy (until Feb 1970)		Esophagoscopy: changes in the lower esophagus Hb: 9.1 g% Weight: 3rd percentile Height: 3rd percentile
	Jan 1971	Stenosis disappeared		
	Nov 1972	Severe reflux esophagitis; anemia Fundoplication; plication of diaphragm Pyloromyotomy; bougienage Gastrostomy (until Jan 1973)		
	Nov 1974	Severe distal esophagitis Regular bougienage (last in Dec 1977)		

Complaints

Twelve parents said that their children had still some complaints after discontinuation of the therapy. Seven still vomited, five had difficulties in swallowing, four were constipated, three had diarrhea, two had recurrent infections of the upper respiratory tract, one had a poor appetite, and one had heartburn.

Follow-up Examination

The following children were asked to appear for a follow-up examination:
- Children who after discontinuation of the therapy or after discharge from hospital still had some complaints
- Children without symptoms but where the parents wished a follow-up examination

The follow-up examination consisted in the taking of an exact clinical history, clinical examination, hemoglobin examination, and measurement of height and weight. Routine radiographic control was not carried out unless there were special indications.

Results in Children Without Symptoms Examined Because the Parents Wished It

Six children were examined. These children are all healthy. They had no complaints at the time of examination. Height and weight were within normal limits.

Results in Children with Complaints After Discontinuation of Therapy or After Discharge from Hospital

In 12 children the parents stated in reply to the questionnaire that there were still some complaints. At the time of examination, the hemoglobin was normal. Only one of the children who had suffered from neonatal asphyxia and epilepsy had a weight under the 3rd percentile.

One child suffered from diarrhea and flatulence, which may have been the result of the surgical treatment (fundoplication, pyloroplasty, and vagotomy). This child's weight and hemoglobin were normal.

At the time of the examination, four children were not cured. The details can be seen from Table 7.

Discussion

Diagnosis of hiatus hernia should be made as early as possible (Carré 1971; Randolph et al. 1974). In nearly 100% of our patients, vomiting was the leading symptom, occurring soon after birth. Type and frequency of vomiting was very variable and changed in the same patient from time to time. A typical type of vomiting in patients with hiatus hernia cannot be demonstrated. Depending on the severity of the reflux and the duration of the disease, secondary changes, such as esophagitis and anemia, were observed. Anemia was also partly due to the deficient nutrition. This was shown by the fact that an esophagitis could be demonstrated in only 11 of the 19 patients with anemia. According to Boix-Ochoa and Rehbein (1965), the frequency of esophageal stenosis in the lower esophageal segment increases with age and the duration of the reflux. Because of the early diagnosis, there were only two instances of esophageal stenosis among our patients. Similar to the patients described by Lilly and Randolph (1968), 67.7% of our patients were under 6 mon old when first admitted to hospital.

Conforming with other reports in the literature (Carcassone et al. 1974; Follette et al. 1976; Botha 1958), we found a typical combination of hiatus hernia and left-sided operated diaphragmatic eventration as well as cerebral paralysis. The combination of hiatus hernia and pyloric stenosis (Roviralta syndrome) was seen three times (5%). Pellerin et al. (1974) found a gastroesophageal reflux in 13% of their patients with pyloric stenosis. Medical treatment of patients with Roviralta syndrome following pyloromyotomy seems, therefore, indicated in order to prevent reflux esophagitis, which may occur in 38%.

We agree with Vos (1971) that esophageal reflux is a definite indication for therapy, even if radiology cannot definitely demonstrate a hiatus hernia (in our patients, 20 out of 65).

The literature shows that it is impossible to be dogmatic about the type of treatment for children with hiatus hernia. This is partly due to the fact that in an unpredictable percentage of the patients, spontaneous healing occurs (Prinsen 1975; Randolph et al. 1974), and it is difficult to judge the effect of conservative therapy.

One report (Botha 1958) showed that after 2 years without any treatment at all, 65% of the children had no symptoms any more. Several authors state that in approximately 20% of the patients who are clinically healed, the radiological findings have not changed (Lefrançois et al. 1975; Nussle et al. 1969). Carré (1972) reported that healing occurred in 66% of children between 2 and 4 years of age, but only in 20% in children between 10 adn 15 years of age. In a more recent study of the same author (Carré et al. 1977), half of the patients over 20 years of age who were clinically cured still had a hiatus hernia when examined radiologically.

Nevertheless, we are of the opinion that, apart from definite indications for primary operation, conservative treatment should always be tried (Lilly and Randolph 1968; Vos and Boerema 1971).

We agree with Prinsen (1975) that the children should be treated conservatively at first for 2 weeks. Only if conservative treatment is not successful should an operation be considered.

Conservative treatment consisting of a combination of sitting the patient up, thickening of the food, and antacids should be carried out, although Prinsen (1975) and Brown (1963) did not find antacids an advantage. Therapy should be carried out for at least 10 weeks to 3 mon after the symptoms have disappeared, in order to minimize a possible recurrence.

Of our 20 patients with hiatus hernia type 1, only two had to be primarily operated. In two further patients, conservative treatment was unsuccessful, necessitating a fundoplication. Of the 34 patients with type 2, 23 were initially treated conservatively, four without success. Nothing definite can be said about the effect of conservative therapy and the necessity of operations in children with a hiatus hernia *forme majeure* because the number of the patients is insufficient.

Lilly and Randolph (1968) did not find any relationship between the severity of the symptoms and the success of conservative therapy. Conservative therapy appears to be successful in between 63% (Nussle et al. 1969) and 86% of the patients (Sørensen 1967). On a short-term basis a significant relationship between the success of therapy and the radiological findings was observed. In type 1, treatment was successful in 87%, in type 2 in 58%. At present, 83.3% of our patients with type 2 hiatus hernia are definitely without complaints. In a 20-year study carried out by Astley et al. (1977), they showed that after 20 years, 92% of the conservatively treated patients (a total of 86) were without symptoms. Our findings seem to justify primary conservative treatment in cases with hiatus hernia *forme mineure*. We are of the opinion that early operation may be unnecessary in nine out of ten cases.

If conservative therapy is unsuccessful, immediate surgery should be carried out. This was the case in 13% of our patients. This figure seems to be below the average of 15%–28% (Brown 1963; Randolph et al. 1974). Further indications for primary operations are paraesophageal hernias, persistent esophagitis, stenosis of the lower esophagus, and severe physical retardation because of massive vomiting.

The optimal operative therapy is the fundoplication of Nissen. In the years 1966–1976, 24 of the 26 operated children were treated by fundoplication. In four patients, several operations were necessary.

The postoperative results in cases without stenosis are good or very good (Bettex 1974; Bettex and Kuffer 1969; Follette et al. 1976; Genton 1967; Sauvegrain 1957).

Of our patients, 89% were free from symptoms at the time of the follow-up examination. A certain number of the patients complain of a feeling of fullness of the stomach because of difficulties in bringing up swallowed air for a short period after operation. Woodward (1975) states that 54% of the patients complain of this disability. On follow-up examination, only one of our patients was still complaining of this symptom.

Simultaneous vagotomy and pyloroplasty appear not to increase the success rate of operation and should not be carried out routinely (Ellis 1972). Woodward (1975) states that they are associated with an increased morbidity, for instance, the dumping syndrome and diarrhea.

If an esophageal stenosis is present, the success rate of the operation is diminished. It is, therefore, most important that stenoses should be prevented. Stenoses do not depend on the severity of the radiological anomaly (Symposium sur les hernies hiatales de l'enfant 1967). It is noticeable that one of our two patients with a fibrous stricture of the esophagus had a hiatus hernia type 1. Carré (1959) states that 21% of the patients collected from the European literature developed stenoses. Luckily, only two of our 65 patients had an esophageal stenosis.

Summary

Between 1966 and 1976, 65 infants and children were treated because of hiatus hernia. The diagnosis was made radiologically in all cases and in a number of patients endoscopically. 54 patients had a *forme mineure* (types 1 and 2), and 11 had a *forme majeure* (types 3 and 4). Of the 20 patients with type 1, 16 (80%) were successfully treated conservatively; two further patients needed a secondary operation. Of 34 children with type 2, 15 (44%) were treated successfully conservatively, and four needed a secondary operation. Of ten patients with type 3, four (40%) were treated primarily conservatively with success. Two children with type 1, 11 with type 2, six with type 3, and one with type 4 had to be operated on primarily because of severe esophagitis at the time of admission.

From 14 mon to 10 years after discharge from hospital, follow-up examination of 33 patients showed that one child died from another cause. In 14 of the 21 conservatively treated patients and in 12 of the 18 surgically treated patients (66% in both cases), there were no symptoms or complaints. Eight had subjective complaints, but in only four (10.5%) was there a definite complaint. Three of these four patients had associated diseases (spastic tetraplegia, operated jejunal atresia). In these patients, esophagitis was present on follow-up examination and necessitated further treatment.

The treatment of choice for the *forme mineure* without esophagitis should be conservative, and in most cases this will be sufficient. In only a few of these patients did it become necessary to carry out a secondary fundoplication. Operation is indicated primarily in cases with esophagitis and esophageal stenosis as well as in patients with a *forme majeure* of the hiatus hernia.

Résumé

Entre 1966 et 1976, 65 nourrissons et enfants ont été traités pour hernie hiatale (54 cas de forme mineure et 11 cas de forme majeure). Au cours de la première hospitalisation, 20 interventions chirurgicales et 45 traitements médicaux furent pratiqués. Le traitement médical échoua dans 6 cas, entraînant une seconde hospitalisation et une fondoplication selon Nissen.

89,5% des enfants réexaminés de 14 mois à 10 ans après leur hospitalisation étaient guéris. Le traitement médical a donc obtenu la guérison de 85% de formes mineures de hernie hiatale dans le groupe étudié. Il doit donc être le traitement de choix, du moins en ce qui concerne la forme mineure.

Zusammenfassung

Von 65 Kindern, die in den Jahren 1966–1976 im Kinderspital Zürich wegen Hiatushernie „forme mineure“ (54 Fälle) oder Hiatushernie „forme majeure“ (11 Fälle) hospitalisiert waren, wurden im Verlauf der ersten Hospitalisation 20 operativ und 45 konservativ behandelt. In 6 Fällen scheiterte die konservative Therapie, so daß in einer zweiten Hospitalisation eine Fundoplikation nach Nissen notwendig wurde.

Eine Nachkontrolle, 14 Monate bis 10 Jahre nach der Hospitalisation, ergab, daß 89,5% der Kinder definitiv beschwerdefrei waren.

In unserem Patientenkollektiv führte die konservative Therapie bei Hiatushernie „forme mineure“ in 85% zur definitiven Heilung. Sie sollte, abgesehen von eindeutigen Operationsindikationen, immer zuerst versucht werden.

Die Fundoplikation ist in erster Linie bei Mißlingen der konservativen Therapie (keine entscheidende Besserung nach 14tägiger Behandlung) sowie bei den meisten Formen der Hiatushernie „forme majeure“ und bei sekundärer Narbenstenose indiziert.

References

Astley R, Carré IJ, Langmead-Smith R (1977) A 20-year prospective follow-up of childhood hiatal hernia. Br J Radiol 50:400–403

Bettex M (1974) Surgical treatment of hiatus hernia and cardiooesophageal chalasia in infants and children. Paediatrician 3:161–165

Bettex M, Kuffer F (1969) Long-term results of fundoplication in hiatus hernia and cardioesophageal chalasia in infants and children. J Pediatr Surg 4:526–530

Boix-Ochoa J, Rehbein F (1965) Oesophageal stenosis due to reflux oesophagitis. Arch Dis Child 40:197–199

Botha CS (1958) The gastro-oesophageal region in infants. Arch Dis Child 33:78–94

Brown FB (1963) Medical and surgical management of esophageal hiatus hernia in children. Bol Med Hosp Infant Mex 41:17–24

Carcassone M, Grégoire A, Magalon G (1974) Les reflux gastrooesophagiens du nourrisson. Pédiatrie 24:815–924

Carré IJ (1959) The natural history of the partial thoracic stomach ("hiatus hernia") in children. Arch Dis Child 34:344–354

Carré IJ (1971) Conservative management of partial thoracic stomach in children. Paediatr Paedol 6:247–252

Carré IJ (1972) Long-term results of postural treatment in children with a partial thoracic stomach ("hiatus hernia"). Acta Paediatr Scand 61:492–506

Carré IJ, Astley R, Langmead-Smith R (1977) Long-term prospective follow-up of children with hiatal hernia. Gut 18:990

Ellis FH Jr (1972) Esophageal hiatal hernia. N Engl J Med 287:646–649

Follette D, Fonkalsrud EW, Euler A, Ament M (1976) Gastrooesophageal fundoplication for reflux in infants and children. J Pediatr Surg 11:757–761

Genton N (1967) Hernies hiatales: traitement chirurgical par fundoplicature de Nissen chez 62 enfants. Ann Chir Enfant 8:353–359

Lari J, Lister J (1972) Some problems in surgical management of children with hiatus hernia. Arch Dis Child 47:201–206

Lefrançois MC, Jezequel C, Coutel Y (1975) Etude de l-evolution de 43 cas de malpositions oeso-cardio-tubérositaires du nourrisson. Rev Pediatr 11:399–407

Lilly JR, Randolph JG (1968) Hiatal hernia and gastrooesophageal reflux in infants and children. J Thorac Cardiovasc Surg 55:42–53

Nussle D, Genton N, Philippe P (1969) Evolution clinique et radiologique de malpositions cardio-tuberositaires non-operées du nourrisson. Helv Paediatr Acta 24:145–159

Pellerin D, Bertin P, Tovar JA (1974) Reflux gastroesophagien et stenose hypertrophique du pylore. Ann Chir Enfant 15:7–14

Prinsen JE (1975) Hiatus hernia in infants and children: a long-term follow-up of medical therapy. J Pediatr Surg 10:97–102

Randolph JG, Lilly JR, Anderson KD (1974) Surgical treatment of gastroesophageal reflux in infants. Ann Surg 180:479–485

Sauvegrain J (1957) Etude radiologique des malpositions oesophago-cardio-tubérositaires chez le nourrisson et chez l'enfant. 16eme congrès des pédiatres de langue française: rapports 3: 29–42

Sørensen BM (1967) Hiatus hernia in infancy. Acta Paediatr Scand 56:513–521

Symposium sur les hernies hiatales de l'enfant (1967) Ann Chir Inf 8:249–422

Vos A (1971) Gastroesophageal reflux in infants and children. Scand J Gastroenterol 6:369–370

Vos A, Boerema I (1971) Surgical treatment of gastroesophageal reflux in infants and children. J Pediatr Surg 6:101–111

Woodward ER (1975) Sliding esophageal hiatal hernia and reflux peptic esophagitis. Mayo Clin Proc 50:523–527

Immunological and Hematological Consequences of Deficient Function of the Spleen

W. H. Hitzig[1]

Lien: mysterii plenum organum (Galenus)

The following introductory remarks aim at a brief recapitulation of some anatomical and physiological data on the spleen, which might be helpful before the discussion of recent surgical problems with this organ.

Anatomy

The weight of a normal spleen is about one-third of a percent of the body weight (Pearson 1981). The large vessels enter the spleen at the hilus and penetrate together into the trabeculae (Von Möllendorff 1940). Before reaching the splenic pulp, they divide, and the smaller arteries become surrounded by lymphatic tissue, thus forming the central artery of the malpighian body. Subsequently, the artery breaks up into the penicillar arteries, which continue into the contractile capsular arteries, and finally end in the reticulum of the red pulp. This is a network within the cords of Billroth, surrounding the central splenic sinus. The endothelial cells lining both the splenic sinus and Billroth's cords lack a basement membrane,

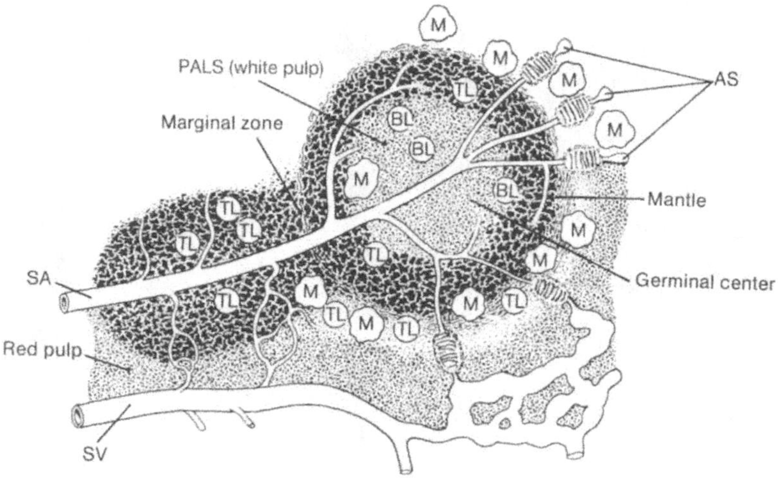

Fig. 1. Structure and function of the spleen. *TL*, thymus-dependent lymphocyte; *BL*, bursa-dependent lymphocyte; *M*, monocyte-macrophage; *SA*, splenic artery; *SV*, splenic vein; *AS*, terminal arteriolar sphincter; *PALS*, periarteriolar lymphocytic sheath. (Craddock et al. 1971)

[1] University Children's Hospital, Steinwiesstr. 75, CH-8032 Zürich/Switzerland

Progress in Pediatric Surgery, Vol. 18
Ed. by P. Wurnig

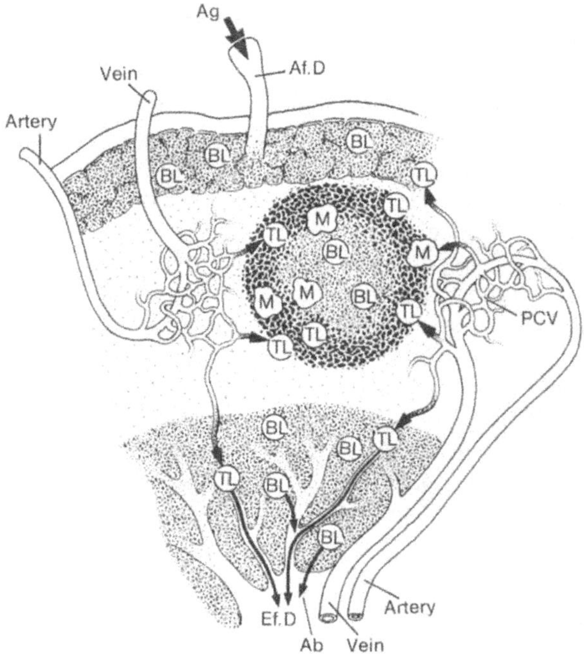

Fig. 2. Structure and function of the lymph node. *BL,* bursa-dependent lymphocyte; *M,* monocyte-macrophage; *Ag,* antigen; *Ab,* antibody; *Af.D,* afferent lymphatic duct; *Ef.D,* efferent lymphatic duct; *PCV,* postcapillary venule. (Craddock et al. 1971)

but they have projections which extend into their respective vascular channels. The potential clefts between the endothelial cells provide an effective filtration system through which red cells and white cells in the Billroth's cord have to pass to regain the splenic sinus and reenter the venous circulation (Pearson 1981).

The white pulp contains numerous T-lymphocytes and macrophages; the germinal centers have in addition, B-lymphocytes, which synthesize specific antibodies (Craddock et al. 1971). A comparison with the structure of a lymph node shows many analogies – the neighborhood of macrophages preparing antigens and lymphocytes making antibodies – but one essential difference: the lymphatic tissue of the spleen is in direct contact with the blood, whereas the afferent limb of the lymph node is exclusively represented by lymph. According to its physiologic functions, the spleen might be designated as "central general lymph node" (Figs. 1 and 2).

Physiology

Some of the mysteries previously associated with the spleen are now replaced by facts: during the embryonal period, the spleen has an important function in hematopoesis; in the postnatal period, it fulfills hematological and immunological functions. Its peculiar structure serves to control every blood cell, which must be squeezed through the endothelial clefts into the venous sinuses. This is accomplished by "culling and pitting," expressions which indicate a selective removal of morphologically abnormal erythrocytes and removal of intraerythrocytic inclusions, such as Howell-Jolly bodies, respectively (Pearson 1981). Rigid cells, like spherocytes or drepanocytes, are retained, phagocytosed, and destroyed. By this mechanism a normal man replaces about 1% of his aged and functionally damaged erythrocytes each day. Foreign blood cells (e.g., introduced by incompatible blood transfusion) or other antigenic material is taken up by macrophages, which transform it into a superantigen and offer it to neighboring lymphocytes. This again exemplifies how intimately the immunological function of the spleen is related with the blood (Craddock et al. 1971; Pearson 1981).

Pathological functions are either hypo- or hypersplenism (Pearson 1981). A person with the first, which may be congenital or acquired, carries the same risks as a splenectomized patient. On the other hand, hypersplenism is characterized by too rapid and too extensive destruction of blood cells, which leads to pancytopenia.

Indications for Splenectomy

In syndromes with hypersplenism (Table 1), there is a clear indication for splenectomy: hemolytic anemias due to rigid erythrocytes are improved by removing the control organ, since erythrocytes now stay in the circulation for a longer time (Schilling 1976). In oncologic diseases the operation has mainly diagnostic value. Sometimes removal of the spleen is necessary for mechanical reasons when removing a tumor, e.g., an infiltrating nephroblastoma. The most important

Table 1. Indications for splenectomy

Hematologic diseases
Spherocytosis, hemoglobinopathy, Wiskott-Aldrich syndrome, thrombocytosis, aplastic anemia
Oncologic diseases
Staging of Hodgkin's disease, lymphomas, tumors in leukemia, nephroblastoma
Immunologic diseases
Autoimmune hemolysis and thrombocytopenia
Infections
Kala-azar, parasites
Syndromes with hypersplenism
Banti's syndrome, splenic vein thrombosis, storage diseases
Trauma
Rupture of the spleen

indication for surgery, rupture of the spleen, until recently was treated by ligation of the hilus and total splenectomy in order to avoid hemorrhage.

Inclination for Infections After Splenectomy

Since 1952 (King and Shumacher 1952) many authors have pointed out increased susceptibility to infections in splenectomized people. This "overwhelming post-splenectomy infection" (OPSI) increases the risk of sepsis, according to extensive collective statistics, by a factor of 58–86 compared with a normal population (Pearson 1981). In patients splenectomized for trauma, the risk for septicemia is increased sixfold, but because of a letal nature of the infections (58%), the risk of death is 200 times greater than in the normal population (Pearson 1981). Micro-organisms found in OPSI are mainly encapsulated bacteria, in half of the cases pneumococci (Table 2). In tropical countries, infections with *Plasmodium malariae* are also frequent.

It is also evident that the nature of the underlying disease for which the patient is operated is important: most unfavorable are malignancies including the spleen; in Hodgkin's disease, though, splenectomy may be compared with a biopsy for staging the extent of the disease.

The development and progress of such an infection in a splenectomized child is extremely rapid with sudden shock and high fever almost without prodromata, and it therefore leads to death within hours. Bacterial cultures in blood and cerebrospinal fluid are positive, and frequently great numbers of free bacteria can be seen in the blood smear.

The reasons for these severe infections are rather well known, as pointed out in the section on physiology. A great number of experimental and clinical work has been done in this field (Craddock et al. 1971; Schwartz et al. 1977). It is obvious that the lack of a normal phagocytic function of the spleen fails to clear infectious material from the circulation. As a consequence, no bacteria can be offered by the phagocytes to macrophages, which in turn should transmit the information on the penetrating antigen to lymphocytes. Normally, within 3–5 days, "early antibodies" of the IgM type would be formed, and these would be

Table 2. Microorganisms found in overwhelming postsplenectomy infections

Pneumococci	49.0%
Escherichia coli	10.9%
Meningococci	10.4%
Hemophilus influenzae	9.3%
Other organisms	10.6%
No organisms found	9.5%

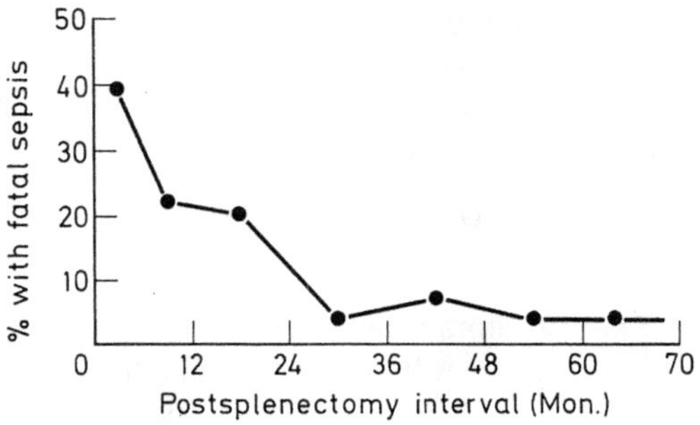

Fig. 3. Incidence of overwhelming postsplenectomy infection as a function of time

replaced gradually by the persisting IgG antibodies (Schwartz et al. 1977). After this lag period the first line of defense represented by the phagocytes could be replaced by the more sensitive antibodies, which opsonize particulate antigen, i.e., "make it palatable" to phagocytes.

These functions can hardly be substituted by the liver, since the blood flow is too rapid to allow phagocytosis of particles which are not heavily opsonized; in addition, the close relationship with lymphatic tissue, of such great importance in the spleen, is lacking in the liver. Most of the OPSI are seen in the first 2 years after splenectomy. Later they also occur but are much rarer (Fig. 3).

Therapy and Prophylaxis

Treatment of OPSI is severely handicapped because of the fulminant course. Antibiotic treatment should be started as quickly as possible. However, prophylaxis of the infections is of far greater importance. There are three possibilities (Table 3):

1. Immunization against pneumococci (Pneumovax) aiming at preparing sufficient amounts of opsonins. This procedure has two limitations: small children (<2 years of age) are unable to form antibodies against pneumococcal polysaccharides, and there is no protection against germs other than pneumococci included in the vaccine.
2. Prophylactic treatment with antibiotics effectively suppressing pneumococci and most of the other microorganisms: for practical reasons amoxicillin (three

Table 3. Prophylaxis of overwhelming postsplenectomy infections

Children <2 years of age:	prophylaxis with amoxicillin or sulfamethoxazole
Children >2 years of age:	pneumococcal vaccination and self-dispensation of amoxicillin or sulfamethoxazole (in reticulo-endothelial system diseases)
All ages:	preservation of spleen in trauma; malaria prophylaxis in tropical countries

times a day) or sulfamethoxazole and trimethoprim (once daily) is recommended.
3. New operative techniques conserving splenic tissue, which is one of the main topics of this monograph (Benjamin et al. 1980; Likhite 1978; Livaditis and Sandberg 1980; Shackford et al. 1981; Tavassoli et al. 1973; Youssef and Stauffer 1982).

Summary

This brief outline of the anatomy and physiology of the spleen points out the intimate relations between blood stream and lymphatic tissue, which enables it to perform many controlling functions: all blood cells are checked and removed, if necessary; antigens are detected, phagocytosed, and offered to the immune system, which reacts by formation of antibodies.

Résumé

Cette brève étude de l'anatomie et de la physiologie de la rate souligne les relations étroites qui existent entre le flux vasculaire sanguin et les tissus lymphatiques, lui permettant d'exercer de nombreuses fonctions de contrôle: toutes les cellules sanguines sont vérifiées et supprimées si nécessaire; les antigènes sont détectés, phagocytés et présentés au système immunitaire qui réagit en formant des anticorps.

Zusammenfassung

Diese kurzen Ausführungen zur Anatomie und Physiologie der Milz betonen die engen Beziehungen zwischen Blutstrom und lymphatischem Gewebe, wodurch viele Kontrollfunktionen ermöglicht werden: alle Blutzellen werden durchgecheckt und, wenn nötig, aus dem Verkehr gezogen, Antigene werden entdeckt, phagozytiert und dem Immunsystem ausgesetzt, das mit der Bildung von Antikörpern reagiert.

References

Benjamin JT, Komp DM, Shaw A, McMillan CW (1978) Alternatives to total splenectomy: two case reports. J Pediatr Surg 13:139

Craddock CG, Longmire R, McMillan R (1971) Lymphocytes and the immune response. N Engl J Med 285:378

King H, Shumacher HB (1952) Susceptibility after splenectomy performed in infancy. Ann Surg 136:239

Likhite VV (1978) Protection against fulminant sepsis in splenectomized mice by implantation of autochthonous splenic tissue. Exp Hematol 6:433

Livaditis A, Sandberg G (1980) Splenic autotransplantation: an experimental study. Z Kinderchir 29:148

Pearson HA (1981) The spleen and disturbances of splenic function. In: Nathan, Oski (eds) Hematology of infancy and childhood. Saunders, Philadelphia London Toronto, p 887

Schilling RF (1976) Hereditary spherocytosis: a study of splenectomized persons. Semin Hematol 13:169

Schwartz AD, Dadash-Zadeh M, Goldstein R, Luck S, Conway JJ (1977) Antibody response to intravenous immunization following splenic tissue autotransplantation in Sprague-Dawley rats. Blood 49:779

Shackford SR, Sise MJ, Virgilio RW, Peters RM (1981) Evaluation of splenorrhaphy: a grading system for splenic trauma. J Trauma 21:538

Tavassoli M, Ratzan RJ, Crosby WH (1973) Studies on regeneration of heterotopic splenic autotransplants. Blood 41:701

Von Möllendorff W (1940) Lehrbuch der Histologie. Fischer, Jena

Youssef S, Stauffer UG (1982) Heterotope Autotransplantation von Milzgewebe nach traumatischer Milzruptur – eine Lösung bei unumgänglicher Splenektomie? Z Kinderchir 35:88

Immunological Consequences of Splenectomy

M. Eibl[1]

Several reports have called attention to the occurrence of overwhelming infection in patients who had undergone splenectomy (Bisno 1971; Editorial 1976; Likhite 1976). While patients who have had splenectomy in infancy and/or for hematological malignancies (Chilcote et al. 1976; Edwards and Digioia 1976; Ein et al. 1977; Klaue et al. 1979) are more likely to develop such infections, mostly caused by pyogenic microorganisms, infections occur in patients splenectomized after trauma as well (Eisenberg et al. 1976; Pringle 1981; Robinette and Fraumeni 1977; Shandling 1976). Information on the function or capacity of the spleen will help to understand why the removal of this organ may lead to these severe complications.

The spleen is the largest individual organ of the phagocytic apparatus with approximately 25% of the body's phagocytic capacity. Aged autologous cells, homologous cells, and other antigens, both soluble and particulate, are eliminated by this system (Saba 1970). Phagocytic cells are the phylogenetically oldest means to recognize nonself. After a particle – an antigen – has been recognized as foreign, it is phagocytosed, processed, and expressed in the membrane of the macrophage in close connection with products of the major histocompatibility locus, i.e., in close connection with self-determinants.

Phagocytic cells have different receptors to interact with the particles to be phagocytosed. The receptors for certain sugars, especially manose, are of great importance for the attachment of bacteria. Such sugars are also present in different cell walls, and the respective receptors seem to represent one of the general recognition sites. When microorganisms are opsonized by IgG antibodies, phagocytes recognize them via their Fc receptor. If opsonization takes place by complement activation, either directly, by activation of the alternative pathway, or antibody-mediated, via the classical pathway, the complement component $C3_b$ remains on the microbial surface and is recognized by $C3_b$ receptors on phagocytes. Phagocytosis by Fc and $C3_b$ receptors is faster and much more efficient than in serum-free environment.

Particles which are minimally or insufficiently opsonized (with low-titer IgG antibody) are preferentially cleared from the circulation by the spleen. An increase in the concentration of opsonizing factors is followed by preferential phagocytosis through the liver (Benacerraf et al. 1959). This implies that the spleen is the most important site of clearance in the early phase of microbial invasion, i.e., before sufficient amounts of specific antibodies are produced and

[1]Institute of Immunology, University of Vienna, Borschkegasse 8a, A-1090 Wien/Austria

Progress in Pediatric Surgery, Vol. 18
Ed. by P. Wurnig

when clearance depends on cross-reacting antibodies, present in low concentrations from previous contacts with other bacterial antigens.

The uptake of particles from the peripheral blood is also the first step in the immune response. Macrophages ingest the bacteria, and the majority of the microorganisms are killed within the phagocytic cell or possibly already in the phase of adherence extracellularly. Part of the antigenic material is processed and re-expressed in the cell membrane, in close proximity to the products of the major histocompatibility complex (MHC). T cells recognize the antigen together with self-determinants and proliferate (Eibl et al. 1982).

As has been shown by several investigators with regard to cells of experimental animals, and as we were able to demonstrate for the human system with *Escherichia coli* as antigen, T cell proliferation is dose dependent in two respects:

1. The higher the dose of antigen ingested, the higher the proliferative response.
2. The macrophage: T cell ratio influences the response as well. Higher proportions of macrophages induce a higher T cell response at the same concentration of antigen (Eibl et al. 1982).

In the case of the splenectomized individuals, the uptake of antigen is significantly lower than in healthy persons, as has been demonstrated with IgG-coated red cells in humans as well as by opsonized pneumococci in splenectomized guinea pigs (Hosea et al. 1981b). One reason for this diminished uptake could be that the anatomical construction of the spleen allows for a longer lasting contact between particulate antigens and phagocytic cells than is the case in other organs. Antigen uptake by the phagocytic cell is strongly dependent on the time of contact between the antigen and the respective phagocyte.

It can be assumed that due to differences in microcirculation the antigen is available for a longer period of time in the spleen than in other organs.

Close physical contact between the antigen-presenting cell and T-lymphocytes is essential in the early phase of the immune response. The spleen provides a favorable site for this interaction because of the large numbers of phagocytic cells surrounded by T cells (Eibl et al. 1982).

The first cells activated by the antigen-presenting macrophage are inducer T cells. They belong to the T4 subpopulation and initiate both the proliferation of helper T cells and the activation of suppressor T cells. Helper T cells are required for the proliferation and differentiation of antigen-reactive B cells. T4 cells are also capable of producing factors called lymphokines, which affect the migration, different effector functions, and bactericidal capacity of macrophages. Immunological reactions are subject to regulation by control mechanisms. The function of this regulatory system is as complicated as the immune response itself and is activated by antigen parallel to immunological effector functions. A series of cells with immune regulatory potential have been identified: macrophages with immunosuppressive function (Miller and Baker 1979) have been demonstrated, especially in connection with infections caused by intracellular microorganisms, for example, acid-fast bacilli. Suppressor T cells are of great importance in the control of antibody production. By using haptens as antigens in the mouse system, a circuit of three cells – TS1, TS2, TS3 – has been identified (Amsbaugh et al.

1978). Each of these cells produces a factor, and as the last stage of sequential activation, a factor is produced which directly suppresses the immune response.

While macrophage-bound antigen mainly induces helper cells, free antigen preferentially stimulates suppression.

Looking at the spleen as the site of a delicate balance between activation of the immune response and its suppression (Amsbaugh et al. 1978; Millard and Banerjee 1979; Romball and Weigle 1977; Roubinian et al. 1977; Rozing et al. 1978) makes the large number of results understandable, which at first sight could have been regarded as contradictory.

In splenectomized patients the number of phagocytic cells is greatly reduced. For this reason less macrophage-bound antigen will be presented to T cells, and large amounts of free antigen will be available. In addition, the ratio between macrophages and T cells will be changed unfavorably. These circumstances will affect antibody production, and it is not surprising that different investigators looking for antibody production in splenectomized patients have found that significantly lower amounts of antibodies are produced, especially against particulate antigens. Jandl and Kaplan (1960) and several other authors demonstrated an impaired response against homologous erythrocytes in splenectomized volunteers, and the Wedgwood group (Sullivan et al. 1978), investigating the immune response to bacteriophage, described an impaired response in splenectomized individuals as well. Of great importance is the diminished production of antibodies for different pneumococci (Giebink et al. 1979, 1980; Hosea et al. 1981a; Passl et al. 1976, 1978; Sullivan et al. 1978; Winkelstein and Lambert 1975) and *E. coli* (Passl et al. 1976, 1978). Both specific antibodies and serum opsonic activity were found deficient in splenectomized individuals (Giebink et al. 1980; Winkelstein and Lambert 1975), but differences in the immune response against different strains of pneumococci are substantial (Giebink et al. 1980). These differences are also responsible for contradictory results from various investigators. Pneumococci of groups 6 and 4 are weak antigens, and defects in splenectomized patients were most common with respect to antibodies against these strains. Type 6 pneumococci have been found responsible in several cases of overwhelming postsplenectomy infections (Giebink et al. 1979). This type is present in the polyvalent pneumococcal polysaccharide vaccine, but it has been found that several splenectomized patients do not respond to it.

Most of the patients who have to be considered as vaccine failures are splenectomized individuals, and the infecting microorganism is mostly type 6 pneumococci. Still pneumococcal vaccination in splenectomized persons is most advisable and should be carried out, irrespective of the time interval to splenectomy.

In serial determinations of serum Ig in groups of splenectomized patients, a lowering of IgM is a general finding (Chilcote et al. 1976; Westerhausen et al. 1981; Winkelmeyer et al. 1981); IgA level is rather increased. Both high and low levels of IgG have been reported. Nitsche et al. (1976) found high levels in the early postoperative phase, Claret et al. (1975) low levels later. Considering the importance of the spleen in immunoregulation, these discrepancies are not surprising.

Cellular immune functions are less well known in splenectomized patients than humoral parameters. A decrease in T cell population (Millard and Banerjee 1979; Westerhausen et al. 1981; Winkelmeyer et al. 1981) with an increase of B cells is probably due to regulatory dysfunctions. There are also indications that the homing of lymphocyte subpopulations is influenced by the spleen and that blood lymphocytes in splenectomized individuals, therefore, show different composition of subsets than in healthy persons. Proliferative responses to mitogens were described as reduced. These findings were more significant shortly after the operation, but could also be detected a long time afterwards (Winkelmeyer et al. 1981).

Our own results (C. Müller, M. Eibl: Manuscript in preparation) indicate that the number of antibody-producing cells is significantly lower in the peripheral blood of splenectomized individuals than in healthy persons. The difference between the two groups was much larger than would have been expected on the basis of Ig and antibody levels, pointing to a differential homing of antibody-producing cells.

It appears likely that antibody-producing cells circulate in higher frequency in healthy persons, while in the splenectomized they migrate and stay in organs like lymph nodes and the bone marrow. Results obtained in experimental animals support this hypothesis.

Conclusion

The functions of the spleen include phagocytosis, participation in antibody production (especially against particulate antigens) and in the primary response, regulation of the immune response and influence on the homing of immunocompetent opsonins (Spirer et al. 1977). The immunological consequences of splenectomy can only be understood if we realize that none of these functions is unique to the spleen, but, on the other hand, that the spleen is an important part of the immune system and its removal will influence immunological functions quantitatively, affecting certain immunological reactions more than others.

Summary

A series of reports have dealt with the occurrence of overwhelming infections in splenectomized patients. Being the largest individual organ of the phagocytic apparatus, the spleen is responsible for the phagocytosis of insufficiently opsonized particles. These are taken up by macrophages, processed, and expressed, together with determinants of the HLA system, on the membrane of the macrophage. T cells recognize these structures and proliferate in response, thus inducing a series of immunoregulatory mechanisms. The anatomic design of the spleen allows for close contact between macrophages and T cells. Thus, splenectomy represents a major intervention into the immunologic system. Splenectomized patients have been shown to have low concentrations of IgM, decreased production of antibodies directed against pneumococci and *Escherichia coli,* and several defects in cellular immune function, including decreased numbers of T cells and a reduction in lymphocyte proliferative responses. Thus, the removal of the spleen affects certain immunological reactions, which are reflected by a number of clinical findings.

Résumé

Un nombre assez important de publications ont étudié la survenue d'infections fulgurantes chez les malades splénectomisés. La rate est le plus grand organe isolé du système phagocytaire et est chargée de la phagocytose des microorganismes insuffisamment opsonisés qui sont absorbés par les macrophages, transformés puis exprimés avec les déterminants du système HLA sur la membrane de ces macrophages. Les cellules T reconnaissent ces structures, se multiplient en réponse et engendrent ainsi les mécanismes de la régulation immunitaire. La structure anatomique de la rate permet aux cellules T et aux macrophages d'être en contact étroit. La splénectomie constitue donc une atteinte grave à l'intégrité du système immunologique. La concentration IgM des patients splénectomisés est abaissée et ils produisent moins d'anticorps contre le pneumocque et l'Escherichia coli. Leur système cellulaire immunitaire est déficient (moins de cellules T et ralentissement de la prolifération des lymphocytes). L'ablation de la rate affecte donc certains mécanismes immunitaires comme en témoigne une série d'observations cliniques.

Zusammenfassung

Eine Anzahl von Publikationen haben das Problem des Auftretens von fulminanten Infektionen bei splenektomierten Patienten zum Thema. Die Milz ist das größte Einzelorgan des phagozytierenden Systems und verantwortlich für die Phagozytose von ungenügend opsonisierten Mikroorganismen. Makrophagen nehmen Antigene auf, verarbeiten sie und exprimieren sie zusammen mit Determinanten des HLA-Systems an ihrer Membran, wodurch T-Zellen, die diese Strukturen erkennen, zur Proliferation und damit zur Induktion immunregulatorischer Mechanismen angeregt werden. Die anatomische Konstruktion der Milz ermöglicht einen engen Kontakt zwischen Makrophagen und T-Zellen. Eine Splenektomie stellt daher einen gravierenden Eingriff in das immunologische System dar: Splenektomierte Patienten weisen niedrige IgM-Konzentrationen, eine verminderte Produktion von gegen Pneumokokken und Escherichia coli gerichteten Antikörpern und Defekte des zellulären immunologischen Systems auf (erniedrigte Zahlen von T-Zellen sowie eine Verminderung der Proliferation von Lymphozyten). Eine Entfernung der Milz betrifft daher gewisse immunologische Mechanismen, deren Modulation ihren Niederschlag in einer Reihe von klinischen Beobachtungen findet.

References

Amsbaugh DF, Prescott B, Baker PJ (1978) Effect of splenectomy on the expression of regulatory T cell activity. J Immunol 121(4):1483–1485

Benacerraf B, Sebestyen MM, Schlossman S (1959) A quantitative study of the kinetics of blood clearance of ^{32}P-labelled *Escherichia coli* and staphylococci by the reticuloendothelial system. J Exp Med 110(1):27–48

Bisno AL (1971) Hyposplenism and overwhelming pneumococcal infection: a reappraisal. Am J Med Sci 262(2):101–107

Chilcote RR, Baehner RL, Hammond D, the Investigators and Special Studies Committee of the Children's Cancer Study Group (1976) Septicemia and meningitis in children splenectomized for Hodgkin's disease. N Engl J Med 295(15):798–801

Claret I, Morales L, Montaner A (1975) Immunological studies in the postsplenectomy syndrome. J Pediatr Surg 10(1):59–64

Editorial (1976) Infective hazards of splenectomy. Lancet I:1167

Edwards LD, Digioia R (1976) Infections in splenectomized patients. A study of 131 patients. Scand J Infect Dis 8:255–261

Eibl M, Mannhalter JW, Ahmad R (1982) Macrophage-lymphocyte interaction in response to a bacterial antigen *(E. coli).* Clin Exp Immunol 47:260–268

Ein SH, Shandling B, Simpson JS, Stephens CA, Bandi SK (1977) The morbidity and mortality of splenectomy in childhood. Ann Surg 185(3):307–310

Eisenberg BL, Andrassy RJ, Haff RC, Ratner IA (1976) Splenectomy in children. A correlative review of indications and complications in fifty patients. Am J Surg 132:720–723

Giebink GS, Schiffman G, Krivit W, Quie PG (1979) Vaccine-type pneumococcal pneumonia. Occurrence after vaccination in an asplenic patient. JAMA 241:2736–2737

Giebink GS, Foker JE, Youngki K, Schiffman G (1980) Serum antibody and opsonic responses to vaccination with pneumococcal capsular polysaccharide in normal and splenectomized children. J Infect Dis 141(3):404–410

Hosea SW, Brown EJ, Burch CG, Berg RA (1981a) Impaired immune response of splenectomised patients to polyvalent pneumococcal vaccine. Lancet I:804–807

Hosea SW, Brown EJ, Hamburger MI, Frank MM (1981b) Opsonic requirements for intravascular clearance after splenectomy. N Engl J Med 304(5):245–250

Jandl JH, Kaplan ME (1960) The destruction of red cells by antibodies in man. III. Quantitative factors influencing the patterns of hemolysis in vivo. J Clin Invest 39:1145

Klaue P, Eckert P, Kern E (1979) Incidental splenectomy: early and late postoperative complications. Am J Surg 138:296–300

Likhite VV (1976) Immunological impairment and susceptibility to infection after splenectomy. JAMA 236:1376–1377

Millard RE, Banerjee DK (1979) Changes in T and B blood lymphocytes after splenectomy. J Clin Pathol 32:1045–1049

Miller CL, Baker CC (1979) Development of inhibitory macrophage (Ø) after splenectomy. Transplant Proc 11:1460

Nitsche D, Thiede A, Zierott G (1976) Postoperative Veränderungen der Immunglobuline nach Splenektomie. Langenbecks Arch Chir 340:213–218

Passl R, Eibl M, Egkher E, Frisee H, Gaudernak T, Neugebauer G, Vecsei W (1976) Splenektomie im Kindesalter aus traumatischer Ursache und ihre Folgen. Wien Klin Wochenschr 88(18):585–588

Passl R, Eibl M, Egkher E (1978) Immunologische Untersuchungen nach Splenektomie im Kindesalter aus traumatischer Ursache. Zentralbl Chir 103:560–566

Pringle KC (1981) Underreporting of postsplenectomy sepsis. Arch Surg 116:1101

Robinette CD, Fraumeni JF (1977) Splenectomy and subsequent mortality in veterans of the 1939–45 war. Lancet II:127–129

Romball CG, Weigle WO (1977) Splenic role in the regulation of immune responses. Cell Immunol 34:376–384

Roubinian JR, Papoian R, Pillarisetty R, Sawada S, Talal N (1977) Immunological regulation of spontaneous antibodies to DNA and RNA. Immunology 33:399–405

Rozing NH, Brons C, Benner R (1978) Effects of splenectomy on the humoral immune system. Immunology 34:909–917

Saba T (1970) Physiology and physiopathology of the reticuloendothelial system. Arch Intern Med 126:1031–1052

Shandling B (1976) Splenectomy for trauma. Editorial. Arch Surg 111:1325–1326

Spirer Z, Zakuth V, Diamant S, Mondorf W, Stefanescu T, Stabinsky Y, Fridkin M (1977) Decreased tuftsin concentrations in patients who have undergone splenectomy. Br Med J II:1574–1575

Sullivan JL, Ochs HD, Schiffman G, Hammerschlag MR, Miser J, Vichinsky E, Wedgwood RJ (1978) Immune response after splenectomy. Lancet I:178–181

Westerhausen M, Wörsdörfer O, Gessner U, De Giuli R, Senn HJ (1981) Immunological changes following posttraumatic splenectomy. Blut 43:345–353

Winkelmeyer M, Littmann K, Thraenhart O, Tichy G, Kuwert EK, Eigler FW (1981) Veränderungen des humoralen und zellulären Immunsystems nach Splenektomie. Klin Wochenschr 59:485–493

Winkelstein JA, Lambert GH (1975) Pneumococcal serum opsonizing activity in splenectomized children. J Pediatr 87(3):430–433

Immunologic Status of Children After Splenectomy

L. NOACK, K. GDANIETZ[1], and G. MÜLLER[2]

To be able to discuss the situation of splenectomized children, we have tried to follow up 56 patients who had been splenectomized at the age of 1.9 to 16 years.

The splenectomy was performed for hemolytic anemia in 28, thrombocytopenia in 11, rupture of the spleen in four, and portal hypertension in eight patients. The time between splenectomy and follow-up investigation was 9 months to 17 years.

Besides clinical examination and special inquiries for attacks of infections, blood samples to determinate IgG, IgM, and IgA were taken. Only 54 blood samples could be examined using the method of Mancini. After statistical evaluation, three mean values of the splenectomized patients were compared with a control group and the significance of the difference was judged by the *t* test (Table 1).

Like other authors, we found a significantly higher value of IgG in asplenic patients. This is explained by the emigration of memory cells of the B type from the spleen, which continue their reproduction after splenectomy. Most investigators have found higher IgA values in asplenic children. We found, on the contrary, the IgA to be lower, but we could not prove this result statistically.

We found IgM, which is very important in childhood in preventing infections, to be significantly lowered ($P<0.05$), corresponding to the findings of other investigators. This is thought to be produced by a feedback mechanism from the high IgG values to the IgM.

In order to find out something about the behavior of IgG after splenectomy in the different underlying diseases, the mean values of our four groups of diseases were compared with control groups (Table 1).

IgG was elevated and IgM was lowered in all four groups. IgA vared, except for Werlhof's disease.

Nearly the same alterations of the immunoglobulins were found in our patients with different diseases.

At the time of follow-up all patients were well. Five are active in sports. Since operation, three children suffer from recurrent severe infections of the upper airways. These had been splenectomized before the 3rd year of life due to hemolytic anemia.

Another patient with Evan's syndrome developed a generalized enlargement of the lymph nodes after splenectomy, which was understood as an autoimmune

[1] Klinik und Poliklinik für Kinderchirurgie im Städtischen Klinikum Berlin-Buch, Karower Straße 11, DDR-1115 Berlin-Buch

[2] Institut f. med. Immunologie d. Bereiches Med. d. Humboldt-Univ. Berlin (Charité)

Progress in Pediatric Surgery, Vol. 18
Ed. by P. Wurnig

Table 1. Behaviour of IgG, IgM and IgA after splenectomy in childhood after different diseases (*t* test)

Diagnosis	*n*	Ig	Concentration (mg/ml)		*t* Test (significance)	
			Patients ($\bar{x}$)	Control group ($\bar{x}$)	5%	1%
Haemolytic anemia	28	IgG	12.33	10.15	s↑	–
		IgA	1.65	1.73	–	–
		IgM	1.19	1.62	–	–
Werlhof's disease	11	IgG	10.70	10.73	–	–
		IgA	1.61	1.91	–	–
		IgM	1.92	1.55	–	–
Rupture	8	IgG	11.64	10.33	–	–
		IgA	1.72	2.08	–	–
		IgM	1.32	1.96	s↓	–
Portal hypertension	7	IgG	11.11	10.05	–	–
		IgA	1.94	1.71	–	–
		IgM	1.64	1.91	–	–

reaction. This was treated by immunosuppressive therapy. Under this regime a pneumococcal meningitis developed; 50% of all infections after splenectomy are due to pneumococci. Since in this case, the infection developed while the patient was receiving immunosuppressive therapy, the cause may not be the splenectomy alone.

In the fifth case of infection after splenectomy – in this case after rupture of the spleen – the patient developed rheumatic fever and endocarditis; tonsillitis, appendicitis, and chronic relapsing pyelonephritis were further complications in this child.

We have compared the Ig values of the five above-mentioned patients who have had infections with those of five other patients who had no complaints or diseases after splenectomy (Fig. 1). The Ig levels of these ten patients did not correlate with their clinical symptoms. Therefore, it seems that a connection between the behavior of the immunoglobulins and the state of health and symptoms of the patients does not exist.

In contrast, a correspondence between postoperative complications and the age of the children at the time of operation is noted, since relapsing infections were observed in children who were splenectomized before their 3rd year of life.

The underlying disease seems to influence the susceptibility for infections. Traumatic disruption of the spleen has the least effect, while loss of the spleen in portal hypertension leads to the highest rate of infection. However, in our material the severest infection was seen after removal of a ruptured spleen, while the group with portal hypertension was free of such complications.

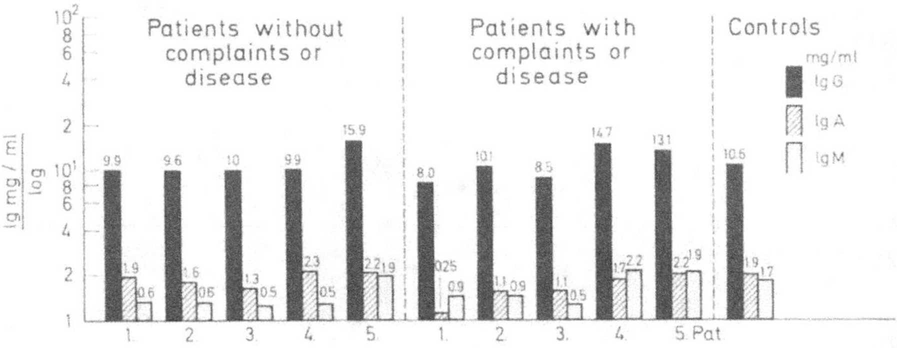

Fig. 1. Comparison of Ig-serum-values of patients without and with postop. complaints or diseases

We had the rare opportunity to observe a child who had undergone a splenectomy on his 1st day of life due to a tumor. Every 2nd month the IgG concentrations were measured. We found that they decreased in the beginning because of disappearance of the maternal antibodies and then rose above normal values. IgM and IgA also rose but never reached normal values. The child, carefully supervised, developed normally and had neither abnormal symptoms nor any diseases. In summary, we must conclude that the susceptibility for infections after splenectomy in childhood cannot be predicted precisely.

Summary

Fifty-six splenectomized children were reexamined to verify their immune status and were compared with a control group. Except for Werlhof's disease, there was a significantly increased serum IgG level in splenectomized children, as compared with the control group, and diminished IgA and IgM levels. Susceptibility to postoperative infections is dependent on age and underlying disease. Generally, susceptibility cannot be predicted following splenectomy in the individual case.

Résumé

56 enfants splénectomisés ont été réexaminés pour vérifier leur état immunitaire et comparés à un groupe de contrôle par rapport auquel on a noté une augmentation significative du niveau des immunoglobulines G chez les enfants splénectomisés; on a egalement noté une diminution des immunoglobulines A et M. La aux infections post-opératoires dépend de l'âge et de la maladie de base. En général, cette réceptivité ne peut pas être prévue en fonction des cas individuels.

Zusammenfassung

56 splenektomierte Kinder wurden auf ihren Immunstatus hin nachuntersucht und mit einer Kontrollgruppe verglichen. Es fand sich eine gegenüber der Kontrollgruppe statistisch signifikant erhöhte Serum-IgG-Konzentration bei den splenektomierten Kindern, während IgA und IgM erniedrigt waren. Die postoperative Infektanfälligkeit ist unabhängig vom Alter und der Grundkrankheit. Insgesamt kann die Infektionsgefährdung nach Splenektomie nicht sicher vorausgesagt werden.

References

Andersen V, Cohn J, Sørensen SF (1976) Immunological studies in children before and after splenectomy. Acta Paediatr Scand 65:409–415

Bürki H, Luscieti P, Pedrinis E, Schädeli J, Hess MW, Cottier H (1974) Milz und Antikörperbildung. Schweiz Med Wochenschr 104:1351–1360

Isa SS, Mirhij NJ, Firzli SS, Slim MS (1974) Postsplenectomy infections in childhood. Z Kinderchir 14:245–251

King H, Shumacker HB (1952) Splenic studies. 1. Susceptibility to infections after splenectomy performed in infancy. Ann Surg 136:239–242

Lennert KA, Kollmar M, Schmidt G (1974) Verhalten der Immunglobuline G, A und M, des Alpha-1-Antitrypsins und Alpha-2-Makroglobulins nach Splenektomie im Kindesalter. Münch Med Wochenschr 115:1979–1994

Matsuyama S, Suzuki N, Namagachi Y (1976) Rupture of the spleen in the newborn: treatment without splenectomy. J Pediatr Surg 11:115–116

Passl R, Eibl M, Egkher E, Frisee H, Gauderna T, Neugebauer G, Vécsei W (1976) Splenektomie im Kindesalter aus traumatischer Ursache und ihre Folgen. Wien Klin Wochenschr 88:585–588

Rauer U, Freund R (1969) Normalwerte von Immunglobulinen im Kindesalter. Monatsschr Kinderheilkd 117:559–563

Walker W (1976) Splenectomy in childhood: a review in England and Wales, 1960–1964. Br J Surg 63:36–43

Ultrasonic Diagnosis of the Spleen

V. Hofmann[1]

As opposed to the liver and the pancreas, in children the spleen is seldom the primary subject of ultrasonic diagnosis. However, it is included incidentally in every sonographic examination of the abdominal area. This discrepancy can be explained by the fact that it is often very difficult to form a clear sonographic picture of the spleen and its pathological changes. The identification of a normal-sized spleen can be difficult in infants and also in older children.

In general, three sections are enough to show the spleen: one longitudinal and two horizontal sections from dorsal and ventral. Normally, the spleen is relatively free of echo and is a sharply confined organ with good sound conduction and a homogenous echo pattern. In contrast with the liver, there are no blood vessels or bile duct sections to be seen, and therefore the picture does not vary.

The first question is the evaluation of spleen size: in splenomegaly the midline is reached or crossed in the horizontal section (Fig. 1). In the vertical section the spleen reaches farther down than the lower pole of the kidney. The most important congenital malformation is the splenic cyst. It is easily recognizable by sonography; other methods of examination, especially invasive ones, are not necessary

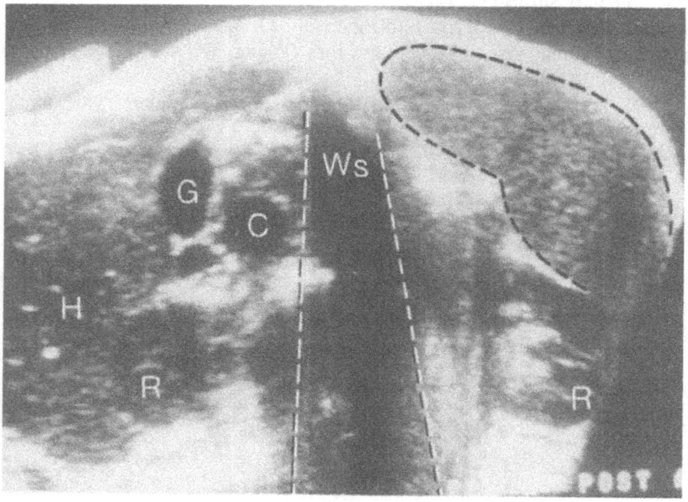

Fig. 1. Horizontal section of epigastrium in splenomegaly. Compound scan technique. *Ws*, vertebral column; *C*, inferior vena cava; *G*, gallbladder; *R*, kidney; *H*, liver

[1] Kinderchirurgische Abteilung St. Barbarakrankenhaus, Halle/Saale, Barbarastr. 3–5, DDR-4020 Halle/Saale

Progress in Pediatric Surgery, Vol. 18
Ed. by P. Wurnig

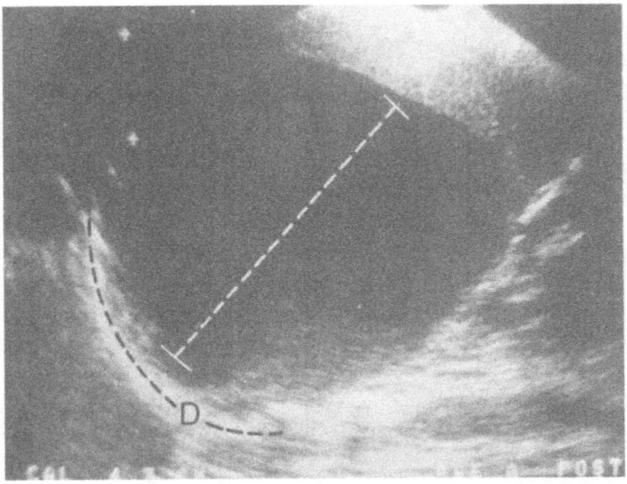

a

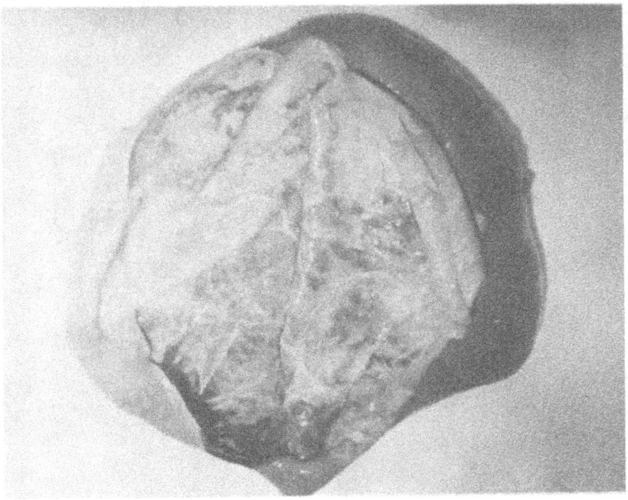

b

Fig. 2a, b. Congenital cyst of the spleen. **a** Longitudinal section, left epigastrium. *D,* diaphragm. **b** Resected specimen

(Fig. 2a, b). In inflammations, it is important to differentiate a subphrenic abscess, a splenic abscess, or a localized abscess in the area of the splenic lodge.

In systemic diseases, the spleen is often the subject of sonographic research. Here it is important above all to recognize pathologic infiltrations by Hodgkin's disease or non-Hodgkin's lymphomas. The structure is noticeably free of echo, and it looks like a cyst with enforced transmission of the sonic beam and dorsal tone increase.

The evaluation of the spleen in blunt trauma of the abdomen is of special interest for pediatric surgeons. Combined with other organic conditions, the effects of a spleen injury can be shown. With constant checks, the formation of a

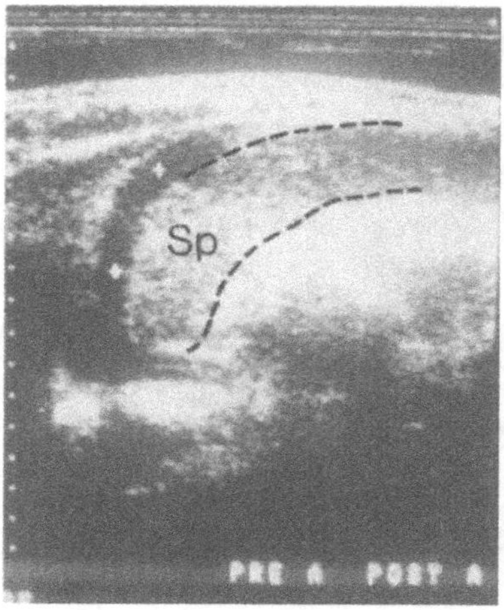

Fig. 3. Small subdiaphragmatic hematoma after trauma to the spleen. *Sp,* spleen

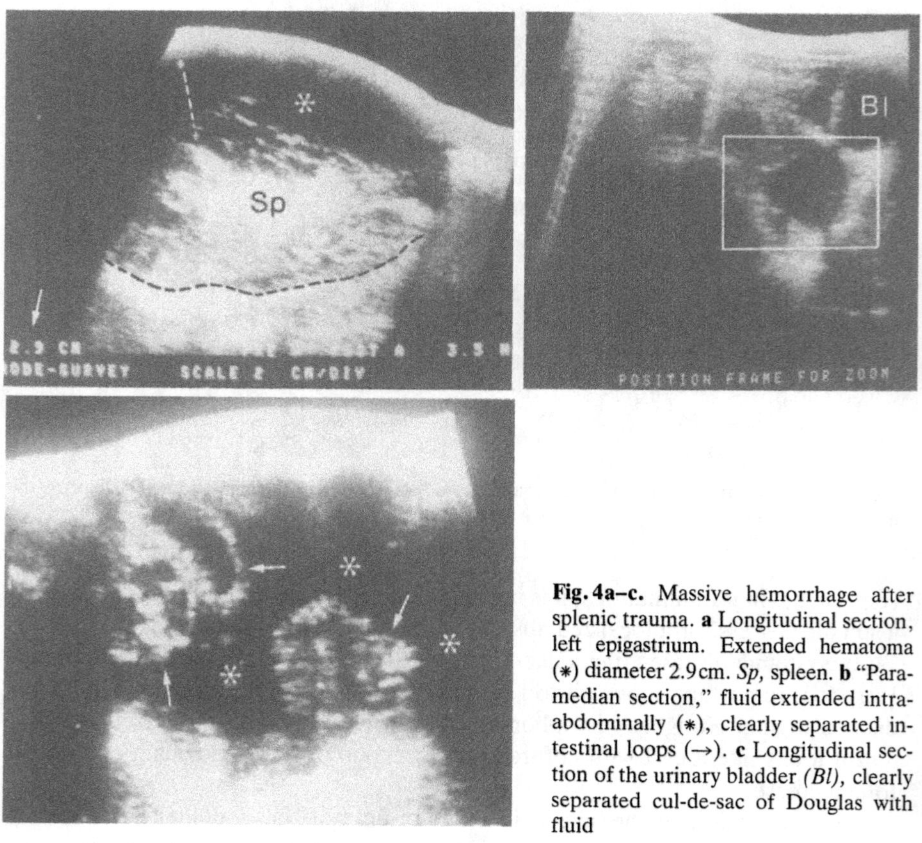

a

c

b

Fig. 4a–c. Massive hemorrhage after splenic trauma. **a** Longitudinal section, left epigastrium. Extended hematoma (∗) diameter 2.9 cm. *Sp,* spleen. **b** "Paramedian section," fluid extended intraabdominally (∗), clearly separated intestinal loops (→). **c** Longitudinal section of the urinary bladder *(Bl),* clearly separated cul-de-sac of Douglas with fluid

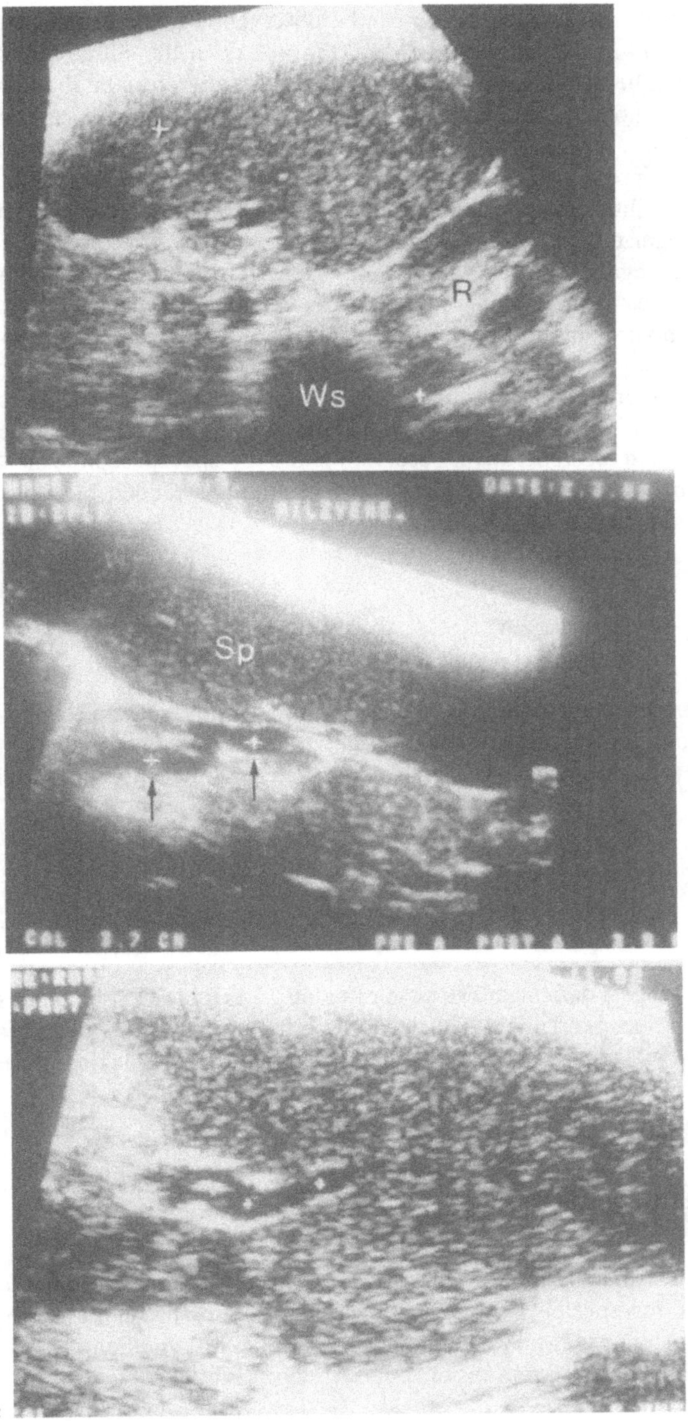

Fig. 5a–c. Splenomegaly in portal hypertension. **a** Horizontal section of epigastrium. The spleen extends beyond the midline. *Ws*, vertebral column; *R*, left kidney. **b** Dilated and twisted (→) splenic vein. **c** Splenic hilus and congestion of the splenic pulp

subcapsular hematoma and its progression can be observed (Fig. 3). In this way the collection of blood in the peritoneal cavity (Fig. 4b) or in the cul-de-sac of Douglas (Fig. 4c) can be demonstrated. Sonography should therefore be the first step in diagnosis and should never be carried out after the lavage. In most cases it can be substituted for a lavage. It is also of great interest to use sonography for follow-up after organ-preserving operations.

Finally, the possibilities for portal hypertension should be presented. Here it is important to recognize the portal vein and its possible changes. It presents as a homogenous splenomegaly (Fig. 5a), but it is important to visualize splenic hilus and changes in the area of the splenic vein (Fig. 5b). In a multiple magnification, the effects of the impaired blood flow in the area of the red pulp can be demonstrated (Fig. 5c).

Summing up, sonography is superior to other diagnostic methods, such as a simple X-ray examination and scintigraphy. Continuous checks for follow-up studies in injuries and postoperative observation are of special significance. Problematic are small ruptures of the parenchyma without extended bleeding, small abscesses, and incipient solid infiltrations.

Summary

The sonographic presentation of the spleen may be difficult and is seldom requested. Main indications for special investigation are traumatic lesions, malignant diseases, such as Hodgkin's or non-Hodgkin's lymphomas, and changes in portal hypertension.

Résumé

Sonographie de la rate est difficile et s'impose rarement. Les indications majeures pour cette investigation particulière sont les lésions traumatiques, les maladies malignes comme la maladie de Hodgkin ou les lymphomes non-Hodgkiniens, et des changements causés par l'hypertension portale.

Zusammenfassung

Die sonographische Darstellung der Milz ist schwierig und selten erforderlich. Hauptindikationen für spezielle Untersuchungen sind traumatische Läsionen, maligne Erkrankungen wie M. Hodgkin und Non-Hodgkin-Lymphome sowie Veränderungen bei portaler Hypertension.

Hematological and Oncological Indications for Splenectomy in Children

C. URBAN[1], M. HÖLLWARTH[2], W. KAULFERSCH[1], and I. SLAVC[1]

The importance of the spleen as an organ of resistance has been shown, and it has been emphasized that the spleen should be preserved whenever possible. Nevertheless, there are indications that in hematologic diseases, the spleen, just because of its increased phagocytic activity, must be removed (Gill 1980; Philippart and Hight 1980).

The most common hematologic indications for splenectomy are:

1. Hemolytic anemia
   a. Membrane defects (spherocytosis)
   b. Hemoglobinopathies
   c. Enzyme defects
   d. Autoimmune diseases
2. Chronic idiopathic thrombocytopenic purpura
3. Hypersplenism

Hemolysis in hereditary spherocytosis can be completely compensated by a splenectomy in most instances. The operation, however, should not be performed before the age of 6 years because of the increased risk of septic complications. The few indications for an earlier splenectomy in cases of hereditary spherocytosis are: frequent blood transfusions, frequent aplastic crises, failure to thrive, and cholestatic jaundice. If there are indications for a splenectomy after the age of 6, ultrasonography can contribute to the decision. If there is no need for transfusion, as in patient with no aplastic crises, splenectomy should only be performed before the age of 10 if gallstones are present. After the age of 10 indications for a splenectomy in uncompensated hemolytic anemia or reticulocytoses are present in more than 50%. For patients with only a slight hemolysis, the splenectomy can be postponed until gallstones appear (Dickerman 1979; Rutkow 1981; Tillmann and Schröter 1982).

The indications for splenectomy in idiopathic thrombocytopenic purpura (ITP) are: acute, dangerous bleeding or thrombocytopenia (below 30 000/mm^3) lasting more than a year along with frequent bleeding. An emergency splenectomy for ITP must be considered if a rapid thrombocyte increase cannot be achieved by other means in the case of critical bleeding (Ahn and Harrington 1977; Mutz and Muntean 1976). In chronic ITP, there is a remission with splenectomy in over 70% of the cases. Recent reports are of interest, according to which the administration of a high intravenous dose of gamma globulin causes a preoperative

[1] Universitäts-Kinderklinik, Auenbruggerplatz 30, A-8036 Graz/Austria
[2] Universitätsklinik für Kinderchirurgie, Heinrichstrasse 31, A-8010 Graz/Austria

Progress in Pediatric Surgery, Vol. 18
Ed. by P. Wurnig

thrombocyte increase by blocking the reticuloendothelial system. This should reduce the risk of complications in the operation for chronic ITP (Ell and Reim 1982; Imbach et al. 1981).

Rarer hematologic indications for splenectomy are chronic and steroid-resistant autoimmune hemolytic anemia and hypersplenism which requires transfusion or leads to bleeding due to thrombocytopenia and which cannot be corrected by other means (e.g., antibiotics for chronic infection). The symptoms for hypersplenism are: splenomegaly, anemia, granulocytopenia, and thrombocytopenia with hyperplasia of bone marrow. Recently alternatives to splenectomy in hypersplenism have been reported, whereby eusplenism is achieved by ligature or partial embolization of the splenic artery (Harouchi et al. 1982; Thanopoulos and Frimas 1982).

Indications for splenectomy in hemolytic anemia due to hemoglobinopathy (e.g., thalassemia) (Isa et al. 1974; Philippart and Hight 1980) or enzyme defects of erythrocytes (e.g., pyruvate kinase deficiency) (Gahr 1981; Schröter and Wonneberger 1976) were not present in our patients.

Splenectomy is indicated in Hodgkin's disease, in splenic tumors, and in cases of splenomegaly associated with systemic malignancies, e.g., chronic myelocytic leukemia. Although at present the staging laparotomy provides the best information about the infradiaphragmatic expansion in Hodgkin's disease, involvement of the spleen can be found in only 30%–40%. In these cases, however, the removal of the spleen offers not only a diagnostic but also a therapeutic advantage because the continuous lymphogenic spread in Hodgkin's disease changes into a hematogenous dissemination via the spleen (Urban et al. 1981). In approximately 65% of the patients who undergo a routine splenectomy during staging laparotomy, the spleen was removed unnecessarily, which must be seen as a disadvantage because of the higher frequency of infection due to the basic disease (Chilcote et al. 1976; Dickerman 1979; Donaldson et al. 1978). In this context, the West German Hodgkin's Therapy Study 1982 is of special interest, since an intraoperative decision strategy for splenectomy was developed: according to the state of the surface of the spleen and the consistency of the lymph nodes at the hilus and along the tail of the pancreas, the conditions inside the spleen are judged; thus, two-thirds of the patients are spared a splenectomy (Schellong et al. 1982).

In systemic diseases, the hypersplenism can become a therapeutic problem and make a splenectomy necessary if the specific treatment of the underlying disease does not lead to a reduction of the splenomegaly (Gill et al. 1981; Gomez et al. 1976).

Results in Our Own Patients

Table 1 shows the 42 patients of the University Children's Clinic in Graz with hematologic and oncologic diseases who were splenectomized during the last 15 years. Main indications for splenectomy were hereditary spherocytosis (14 patients), chronic ITP (11 patients), and Hodgkin's disease (9 patients, one of

Table 1. Diagnosis in patients with splenectomy seen at Children's Clinic, University of Graz, from 1967 to 1982

Hereditary spherocytosis	14
Chronic ITP	11
Hypersplenism	4
Chronic autoimmune hemolytic anemia	1
Hypoplastic anemia	1
Hodgkin's disease	9
Spleen tumors	1
Pseudomalignant immunoproliferation (Canale Smith syndrome)	1

Table 2. Postsplenectomy sepsis in 42 children with splenectomy at Children's Clinic, University of Graz, 1967–1982

Years postoperative	Cases of sepsis	Deaths
<1	2	1
1–2	–	–
2–4	2	1
4–6	–	–
>6	1	–
	5/42 (12%)	2/42 (5%)

whom underwent partial splenectomy). Table 2 shows the postoperative septic complications observed until now. It should be pointed out that patients with an uncomplicated hereditary basic disease, such as hereditary spherocytosis or ITP (under long-term treatment with oral penicillin prophylaxis) had no septic complications. Patients with more serious original diseases requiring splenectomy were affected by septic complications. Two patients with Hodgkin's disease treated by radiation and chemotherapy developed sepsis in the 1st year following splenectomy. The first, a 12-year-old patient, was affected by a *Staphylococcus aureus* sepsis 4 months after the operation and survived, but the second, a 7-year-old child, died from an overwhelming *Staphylococcus albus* sepsis 11 months after operation.

In the 2- to 4-year period following splenectomy, sepsis occurred twice. A 5-year-old patient with systemic lupus erythematosus (an emergency splenectomy for brain hemorrhage was performed under the tentative diagnosis of ITP) survived an *Escherichia coli* sepsis with a kidney abscess under massive antibiotic therapy and a nephrectomy. The second patient, a 17-year-old girl with Hodgkin's disease, stage IVB in the final stage and secondary myelocytic leukemia, died from pneumococcal meningitis (Urban et al. 1981).

In the observation period 6 years after splenectomy, a 23-year-old patient with pseudomalignant immunoproliferation (Kellerer and Mutz 1976) (splenectomy for suspected Hodgkin's disease) survived a pneumococcal meningitis with pneumococcal sepsis. This patient had no regular antibiotic prophylaxis.

Conclusion

Although today surgical methods for preservation of the spleen are of great importance because of the risk of postsplenectomy sepsis, there are still indications for surgery in hematologic and oncologic diseases. In these cases, all methods for organ preservation should be applied because of the limited effects of infection prevention in individual cases.

A splenectomy should also be postponed as long as possible. Preoperatively, a pneumococcal vaccination should be performed and long-term antibiotic prophylaxis should be carried out postoperatively (penicillin, co-trimoxazole) (Dickerman 1979; Philippart and Hight 1980; Stögmann and Paky 1980; Wündisch 1980).

Because of the higher risk of sepsis after splenectomy in Hodgkin's disease, it should be especially considered whether the advantage of a more accurate diagnosis by splenectomy outweighs the higher risk of sepsis, whether a diagnostic hemisplenectomy should be performed, or even if a noninvasive splenic diagnosis by inspection only during a staging laparotomy, preventing the risk of postsplenectomy sepsis (Boles et al. 1979; Editional 1976; Schellong et al. 1982) is sufficient.

Summary

The most common hematologic and oncologic indications for splenectomy in childhood are hereditary spherocytosis, chronic idiopathic thrombocytopenic purpura, hypersplenism, and Hodgkin's disease. Because of the increased incidence of septic complications after splenectomy, benefits to be gained from the operation should be weighed against the risks. A retrospective study was done on the charts of 42 consecutive children with hematologic and oncologic disorders, who underwent splenectomy between 1967 and 1982. The incidence of septic complications after splenectomy was 12%; sepsis, however, only occurred in patients with severe underlying diseases (three patients with Hodgkin's disease, one patient with systemic lupus erythematosus, and one patient with chronic pseudomalignant immunoproliferation). In contrast, none of the patients who were splenectomized for other reasons (mainly hereditary spherocytosis and chronic immune thrombocytopenic purpura) had a septic complication. Two patients with end-stage Hodgkin's disease (5%) experienced fatal septic complications. Although splenectomy is well established for diagnostic and therapeutic considerations in patients with Hodgkin's disease, not all of them might benefit from this operation, and studies with a more limited approach to splenectomy might prove to be of the same therapeutical value.

Résumé

Les indications les plus fréquentes de splénectomie chez l'enfant relèvent de l'oncologie et de l'hématologie: sphérocytose héréditaire, purpura thrombocytopénique chronique, hypersplénisme et maladie de Hodgkin. Avantages et risques de l'intervention doivent être très sérieusement soupesés, le risque septique étant considérable après l'intervention. On a constaté par analyse rétrospective un pourcentage de complications d'ordre septique de 12% chez 42 enfants splénectomisés pour affections relevant de l'hématologie ou de l'oncologie entre 1967 et 1982. Toutefois une septicémie ne survint que dans le cas des patients très gravement affectés (3 patients avec maladie de Hodgkin, un patient présentant un lupus erythémateux systémique et un patient avec prolifération pseudomaligne immunitaire chronique). Par contre, il n'y a eu aucune complication septique chez les autres malades splénectomisés pour d'autres raisons: sphérocytose héréditaire et purpura thrombocytopénique immuno-allergique chronique le plus souvent. La septicémie se révéla fatale dans le cas de 2 patients (5%) atteints de la maladie de Hodgkin au stade terminal. Bien que la splénectomie soit une méthode bien établie dans le cadre diganostique et thérapeutique de la maladie de Hodgkin, il se peut fort bien qu'elle ne convienne pas dans tous les cas et que les thérapeutiques faisant moindre cas de la splénectomie soient tout aussi efficaces.

Zusammenfassung

Die häufigsten hämatologischen und onkologischen Indikationen für die Splenektomie bei Kindern sind hereditäre Sphärozytose, chronische immunallergische thrombozytopenische Pupura, Hypersplenismus und M. Hodgkin. Wegen des erhöhten Risikos von septischen Komplikationen sollten jedoch die Vorteile dieser Operation gegen die Nachteile abgewogen werden. Mittels einer retrospektiven Analyse wurde eine septische Komplikationsrate von 12% an 42 splenektomierten Kindern mit hämatologischen und onkologischen Erkrankungen im Zeitraum 1967–1982 gefunden. Eine Sepsis trat jedoch nur bei Patienten mit schwerer Grundkrankheit (3 Patienten mit M. Hodgkin, 1 Patient mit systemischem Lupus erythematodes und 1 Patient mit chronischer pseudomaligner Immunproliferation) auf. Im Gegensatz dazu kam es bei keinem der aus anderen Gründen splenektomierten Patienten (hauptsächlich Patienten mit hereditärer Sphärozytose und chronischer immunallergischer thrombozytopenischer Purpura) zu einer septischen Komplikation. Bei 2 Patienten (5%) mit M. Hodgkin im Finalstadium endete die Sepsis tödlich. Obwohl die Indikation zur diagnostischen und therapeutischen Splenektomie beim M. Hodgkin gut etabliert ist, profitieren möglicherweise nicht alle Patienten von diesem Eingriff. Hodgkin-Therapiestudien mit begrenzter Splenektomieindikation sind unter Umständen mindestens genauso wirksam.

References

Ahn YS, Harrington WJ (1977) Treatment of idiopathic thrombocytopenic purpura (ITP). Ann Rev Med 28:299–309

Boles ET Jr, Haase GM, Hamoudi AB (1979) Partial splenectomy in staging laparotomy for Hodgkin's disease: an alternative approach. J Pediatr Surg 13:581–586

Chilcote RR, Baehner RL, Hammond D (1976) Septicemia and meningitis in children splenectomized for Hodgkin's disease. N Engl J Med 295:798

Dickerman JD (1979) Splenectomy and sepsis: a warning. Pediatrics 63:938–939

Donaldson SS, Glatstein E, Vosti K (1978) Bacterial infections in pediatric Hodgkin's disease: relationship to radiotherapy, chemotherapy and splenectomy. Cancer 41:1949–1958

Anonymous (1976) Infective hazards of splenectomy. Editorial. Lancet 1:167–168

Ell C, Reim E (1982) Hochdosierte Immunglobulin-Therapie bei chronischer idiopathischer thrombozytopenischer Purpura. Dtsch Med Wochenschr 107:1211–1212

Gahr M (1981) Erythrozytenenzymdefekte – Klinik und Pathophysiologie. Monatsschr Kinderheilkd 129:444–453

Gill FM (1980) Hematologic indications for splenectomy in pediatrics. Am J Pediatr Hematol Oncol 2:41–52

Gill PG, Souter RG, Morris PJ (1981) Splenectomy for hypersplenism in malignant lymphomas. Br J Surg 68:29–33

Gomez GA, Sokal JE, Mittelman A, August CW (1976) Splenectomy for palliation of chronic myelocytic leukemia. Am J Med 61:14–22

Harouchi A, Benchemsi N, Benouhoud M (1982) La ligature de l'artere splenique d'indication hematologique chez l'enfant. Chir Pediatr 23:109–113

Imbach P, D'Apuzzo V, Hirt A, Rossi E, Vest M, Barandun S, Baumgartner C, Morell A, Schöni M, Wagner HP (1981) High dose intravenous gammaglobulin for idiopathic thrombocytopenic purpura in childhood. Lancet 1:1228–1231

Isa SS, Mirkij NJ, Firzli SS, Slim MS (1974) Post-splenectomy infections in childhood. Z Kinderchir 14:245–251

Kellerer K, Mutz I (1976) Chronische pseudomaligne Immunproliferation (Canale-Smith-Syndrom). Eur J Pediatr 121:203–213

Mutz I, Muntean W (1976) Intrakranielle Blutung bei idiopathischer thrombozytopenischer Purpura (ITP). Klin Pädiatr 188:548–551

Philippart AI, Hight DW (1980) Splenectomy in childhood. Altered concepts of management. Am J Pediatr Hematol Oncol 2:61–68

Rutkow IM (1981) Twenty years of splenectomy for hereditary spherocytosis. Arch Surg 116: 306–308

Schellong G, Waubke AK, Langermann HJ, Breu H, Kuhne B, Riehm H, Ritter J (1982) Bedeutung klinischer und intraoperativer Befunde für die Voraussage eines Milzbefalls beim Morbus Hodgkin im Kindesalter: Eine retrospektive statistische Analyse bei 154 Patienten der Therapiestudie HD 78. Klin Pädiatr 194:242–250

Schröter W, Wonneberger B (1976) Klinik und Biochemie des Pyruvatkinasemangels. I. Klinische und hämatologische Untersuchungen. Monatsschr Kinderheilkd 124:1–8

Stögmann W, Paky F (1980) Postsplenektomiesepsis. Pädiatr Praxis 23:429–433

Thanopoulos BD, Frimas CA (1982) Partial splenic embolization in the management of hypersplenism secondary to Gaucher disease. J Pediatr 101:740–743
Tillmann W, Schröter W (1982) Erythrozytenrheologie und Indikation zur Splenektomie bei kongenitalen hämolytischen Anämien. Monatsschr Kinderheilkd 130:254–266
Urban C, Hackl A, Kurz R, Becker H, Mutz I (1981) Probleme des Morbus Hodgkin im Kindesalter. Onkologie 4:331–341
Wündisch GF (1980) Antibiotische Prophylaxe nach Milzexstirpation. Pädiatr Praxis 23:433–434

Selective Hemisplenectomy for Hodgkin's Disease

A. M. Holschneider[1], U. Löhrs, R. Haas, R. Dickerhoff, and W. Gollmitzer[2]

Introduction

The staging laparotomy was introduced in the diagnosis of Hodgkin's disease in 1969 by Glatstein as an exploratory laparotomy with a splenectomy. It allows a more exact analysis of the spread of the disease, which in children leads to a change in the classification of the stage in 15%–20% of the cases, whereby two-thirds of the patients must be classified as higher stages (Hellmann 1974; Lanzowsky et al. 1975; Filler et al. 1975; Cohen et al. 1977; Begemann and Theml 1978; Janka et al. 1978). Involvement of the spleen, which cannot be recognized with clinical methods, is mostly responsible for this. Generally, in both children and adults, the spleen is affected in approximately 30%–50% of cases. Thus, the staging laparotomy has direct influence on the manner and intensity of the therapy. Apart from that, it does not have any therapeutic value (Ihde et al. 1976; Begemann 1975; Begemann and Theml 1978). Also, the occasionally suggested bilateral oophoropexy does not seem to make much sense, as scattered X-rays cannot be avoided. The marking of a possible tumor bed with silver clips has the advantage of facilitating precise, postoperative radiotherapy, but silver clips cause artifacts in later computer tomograms and could thus make the diagnosis of a recurrence more difficult. The clips should be inserted only briefly for an intraoperative X-ray film and removed afterwards before the peritoneum is closed. It is generally regarded as useful to make a thorough diagnosis of splenic involvement so as to avoid not only prophylactic spleen radiation, which could lead to sclerosis and malfunction of the organ, but also the simultaneous radiation of the left kidney and the left lower lobe of the lung.

Dangers of the Staging Laparotomy with Unselected Splenectomy

The staging laparotomy is an operation of medium difficulty, and although the mortality rate is below 1%, there are postoperative complications in 5%–10% of the cases, e.g., abscesses, fistulas, unsatisfactory healing of the wound, bleeding, and pleuritis (Holschneider et al. 1982). In 14.8 of the cases, severe infections can

[1] Kinderchirurgische Klinik im Städt. Kinderkrankenhaus, Amsterdamerstr. 59, D-5000 Köln 60
[2] Kinderchirurgische Klinik der Univ.-Kinderklinik München, Lindwurmstr. 4, D-8000 München 2

Progress in Pediatric Surgery, Vol. 18
Ed. by P. Wurnig

be observed. Kögelmeier found in 1255 children's cases collected from the literature that 3.4% had a severe pneumococcal infection and 2.5% had septicemia.

Fatal outcome was observed in 58% with sepsis and in 22% with meningitis (Kögelmeier 1982). In addition, if a splenectomy is performed habitually and without regard for obvious pathology, a healthy organ is removed 60%–65% of the time. This is all the more serious in Hodgkin's disease because the post-operative complications due to infection are extremely frequent (Mufson 1981).

Selective Complete Splenectomy, According to Schellong

The disadvantages of splenectomy generally performed in Hodgkin's disease convinced Schellong in 1982 to advise selective splenectomy. The spleen is only removed in case of visible changes, as the likelihood of the presence of malignancy here is about 95% (Table 1): 13% of patients belong to this group. Splenectomy is also performed if lymph nodes at the splenic hilus or near the tail of the pancreas are involved macroscopically. In 61% of these patients, or 23.4% of the total, splenic involvement is to be assumed. The spleen is left in place if its appearance is inconspicuous and the pancreatic tail looks normal. This is the case in 63.6% of all patients. Thus, the chance of splenic involvement here is 19.4%.

Splenic involvement can further be reduced by histologic examination of the biopsies. Schellong's investigations have shown that in case of an involvement of abdominal lymph nodes, generally the spleen will also be involved in 80%–91%.

If the abdominal nodes are uninvolved, there is still a 16%–31% chance of splenic involvement.

Schellong's differential approach saved two-thirds of the patients from being splenectomized, which is a great achievement when compared with the general splenectomy of former times. Although in 10% of the cases the spleen is removed without being involved, in 6% of patients the spleen is left in place in spite of being involved, and in a further 3%–4% of children, the spleen is irradiated without being involved. There is an overall misjudgement in about 19%–20% of patients. This could probably be changed by hemisplenectomy. This approach has been advised by Bols in 1967 and was discussed by Schellong in his above-cited paper as an alternative (Schellong et al. 1982).

Table 1. Selective splenectomy, according to Schellong (1982)

Findings	Probability of splenic involvement	Therapy
Surface of spleen alterated	95%	Splenectomy
Lymph nodes at splenic hilus and tail of pancreas involved	60%	Splenectomy
Normal spleen lymph nodes and tail of pancreas normal	19%	No splenectomy

Our Results

In order to find out to what degree a hemisplenectomy is suitable to detect infiltrations of Hodgkin's disease, we reevaluated all lymph nodes, liver biopsies, and spleens which had been removed during staging laparotomies at our unit in the years 1970–1978. They were serially sectioned for histologic examination.

Histology

Out of 25 specimens, five (20%) showed a form of lymphocytic predominance, two (8%) were of the nodular sclerosing type, and 18 (71%) of the mixed cellularity type. In none of the cases did we find a lymphocytic depletion-type of Hodgkin's disease.

Classification

According to the Ann Arbor classification, three (12%) of the cases belonged to stage Ia, nine (36%) to IIa, eight (32%) to IIb, three (12%) to IIIa, one (4%) to IIIb, and one (4%) to IVb. The staging laparotomy meant a change from one stage to another in 11 patients (44%). Ten patients were classified as stage III instead of stage II, and one as stage IV instead of stage III (Table 2).

Splenic Involvement

Of the 25 examined spleens, 14 (56%) showed an infiltration; three (21%) had single nodules with a diameter of over 1 cm (one patient) and under 1 cm (two

Table 2. Change of stage after staging laparotomy

Pre-operative stage	*N*	Post-operative stage	*N*	Reason for change in stage
I	3	I	3	None
II	17	II	7	None
		III	10	Involvement of spleen and lymph nodes not recognized by clinical staging
III	4	III	3	None
		IV	1	Involvement of liver not recognized preoperatively
IV	1	IV	1	None

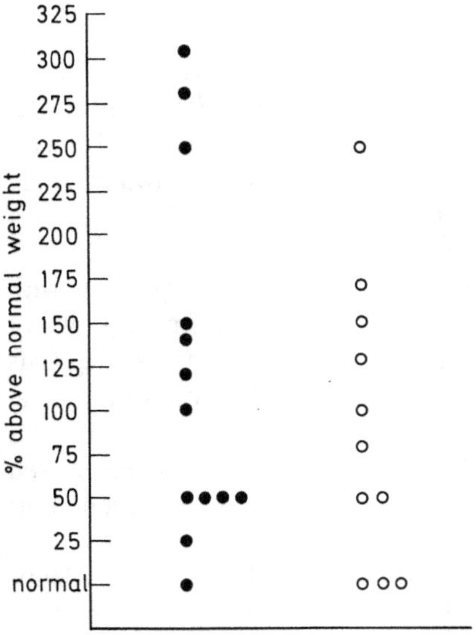

Fig. 1. Weight of spleens affected *(filled circles)* and unaffected *(open circles)* by lymphogranulomatous disease in 25 children

Table 3. Incidence of splenic involvement dependent on microscopic involvement of hilar and pancreatic tail lymph nodes

	Histologic involvement	Number of patients	
		with splenic involvement	without splenic involvement
Lymph nodes at splenic hilus involved	9	9	0
Tail of pancreas not involved	2	1	1

patients). A disseminated infiltration was detected in 11 patients (79%), two of whom had nodules of more than 1 cm, and nine of whom had nodules of less than 1 cm. There was no conclusive difference in weight between spleens affected by Hodgkin's disease and those free of disease.

We found enlarged spleens without infiltrations as well as diseased organs of normal weight (Fig. 1). There was a stronger correlation between involvement of spleen and lymph nodes at the splenic hilus and the tail of the pancreas in our patients than in those of Schellong (1982). All patients with affected lymph nodes in those sites also had an involvement of the spleen.

If the lymph nodes were free of disease, which was the case twice, there was still a possibility for the spleen to be affected (once) (Table 3). In Schellong's much larger series of 105 patients without affected portal nodes, there were still 25 (24%) diseased spleens identified.

Discussion

According to our investigations, we may say that when the spleen is focally affected, an under-staging is possible if a selective hemisplenectomy is done, but still the rate of misinterpretation is lower than in total splenectomy. We found single nodes in only three patients; one node measured 2 × 5 cm, and the other two spleens showed small nodular focal infiltrations.

Surprisingly, the large node had not been palpable. Two of the patients with focal disease showed no involvement of abdominal lymph nodes. In those two of 25 patients (8%), i.e., two of 14 affected organs (14.3%), and exact diagnosis would probably not have been possible by hemisplenectomy because of the focal type of invasion. In Dearth's series (Dearth et al. 1978) of 112 cases, there was localized, small nodular disease in 14 (11.6%), which might have been missed with a hemisplenectomy. Thus, a misinterpretation of 4.1% would be given in his series.

Following our own results as well as those of Dearth (1978), which are identical, we have adopted Schellong's suggestion (1982) since the beginning of 1982 and perform a selective hemisplenectomy instead of a selective splenectomy in connection with the staging laparotomy for Hodgkin's disease (Table 4). Again, according to Schellong, we do a total splenectomy in case of a visible or palpable involvement of the spleen. A hemisplenectomy is carried out if the hilar lymph nodes or those near the tail of the pancreas are macroscopically involved. Frozen sections can help to identify small, focal infiltrations and thus allow removal of the second half of the spleen during the same operation. The organ is left in place if neither the abdominal lymph nodes nor liver or spleen show visible infiltrations.

Only 19 of 98 patients of this group had involvement of the spleen, according to Schellong. In ten of these patients, an involvement of abdominal lymph nodes was demonstrated by histological exmaination. An irradiation of the spleen was applied in these cases. Only nine children remained untreated by irradiation, in spite of involvement of the spleen. One might conclude that it would be advisable to carry out a hemisplenectomy also in those patients whose spleens seem to be unaffected as well as the lymph nodes at the splenic hilus and pancreatic tail.

As we know from numerous investigations (Holschneider et al. 1982), half of the total splenic tissue is sufficient to carry out all immunological tasks of the

Table 4. Indications for splenectomy and hemisplenectomy

Visible involvement of spleen	Splenectomy
Involvement of lymph nodes at splenic hilus and tail of pancreas	Hemisplenectomy → frozen section → splenectomy
Normal spleen and abdominal lymph nodes unaffected	Hemisplenectomy

organ. We do not know, however, whether or not this would be the case also under immunosuppressive therapy with cytotoxic agents. Having this in mind, it seems more reasonable not to perform a hemisplenectomy in patients without visible involvement of lymph nodes and spleen in order not to unnecessarily remove half of a healthy organ in 79 patients. In case of questionable findings, there is still the possibility of taking biopsies from the upper and lower poles of the spleen after having inserted U stitches. The wounds can be closed with the help of human fibrinogen glue. One must keep in mind that according to investigations of Coleman et al. (1982), the irradiation of the spleen leads to fibrotic changes of the organ, which means loss of its immunologic function. In consequence, an irradiated spleen must be considered as immunologically nonexistent and the patient must be treated with antibiotic prophylaxis for 3 years and a pneumococcal vaccination (Belohradsky et al. 1982).

Hemisplenectomy has been carried out by us routinely for 2 years now, having been reserved for solitary diseases of the spleen, like cysts or trauma, in the beginning. Hemisplenectomy is not much more difficult or time-consuming than a splenectomy. By meticulous preparation of the splenic vessels, exact position of the U stitches in the parenchyma, and use of an infrared coagulator or human fibrinogen glue in connection with a collagen sheet, postoperative hemorrhages can be avoided. Since 1982, we have also used hemisplenectomy in three cases of Hodgkin's disease with no postoperative problems. In two cases without pathological intraabdominal findings and without visible changes of the spleen, we could defect microscopic infiltrations of the organ by hemisplenectomy.

Summary

Schellong's recommendation to do a selective splenectomy in Hodgkin's disease supported by our retrospective histological findings in biopsies of lymph nodes and spleens of 25 patients. In addition, we recommend a hemisplenectomy instead of a splenectomy in cases of involvement of the lymph nodes at the pancreatic tail and at the hilus of the spleen. Hemisplenectomy, which is not a more difficult or more time-consuming operation, provides more security in judging an invasion of the spleen.

Résumé

Les résultats de l'étude histologique restrospective des biopsies de ganglions lymphatiques et de la rate de 25 patients atteints de la maladie de Hodgkin sont, de l'avis des auteurs, entièrement en faveur de la splénectomie sélective préconisée par Schellong. Ils recommandent en outre, en cas d'envahissement de ganglions lymphatiques au niveau de la queue du pancréas et dans le hile de la rate, de pratiquer plutôt une hémisplénectomie qui n'est ni beaucoup plus difficile, ni beaucoup plus longue qu'une splénectomie complète mais qui permet d'apprécier plus exactement l'extension tumorale à la rate.

Zusammenfassung

Anhand der retrospektiven histologischen Untersuchung von Lymphknotenbiopsiematerial sowie der Milz bei 25 Patienten mit M. Hodgkin wird der Vorschlag Schellongs zur selektiven Splenektomie unterstrichen. Darüber hinaus wird empfohlen, da die Hemisplenektomie keinen die Operation wesentlich erschwerenden und verzögernderen Eingriff darstellt, jedoch eine größere Sicherheit in der Beurteilung eines fraglichen Milzbefalles mit sich bringt, bei positivem Befall von Pankreasschwanz- und Milzhiluslymphknoten statt der Splenektomie eine Hemisplenektomie durchzuführen.

References

Begemann H (1975) Die Splenektomie beim Lymphogranulomatose-Kranken. Med Klinik 70:591

Begemann H, Theml H (1978) Zur Frage der Splenektomie bei Lymphogranulomatose. Klinikarzt 7:714

Behloradsky BH, Däumling S, Roos R, et al (1982) Postsplenektomie-Infektionen und Pneumokokkenimpfung im kinderchirurgischen Bereich. Z Kinderchir 35:140

Cohen IT, Higgins GR, et al (1977) Staging laparotomy for Hodgkin's disease in children. Arch Surg 112:948

Coleman CN, McDougall IR, et al (1982) Functional hyposplenia after splenic irradiation for Hodgkin's disease. Ann Intern Med 96:44

Dearth JC, Gichrist G, et al (1978) Partial splenectomy for staging Hodgkin's disease: risk of false-negative results. N Engl J Med 299:345

Filler RM, Jaffe N, et al (1975) Experience with clinical and operative staging of Hodgkin's disease in children. J Pediatr Surg 10:321

Glatstein E (1969) The value of laparotomy and splenectomy in the staging of Hodgkin's disease. Cancer 24:709

Hellmann S (1974) What laparotomy has brought. N Engl J Med 290:894

Holschneider AM, Däumling S, Strasser B, et al (1982) Erfahrungen mit der heterotopen Autotransplantation von Milzgewebe im Kindesalter. Z Kinderchir 35:145

Ihde DC, De Vita VT, et al (1976) Effect of splenectomy on tolerance to combination chemotherapy in patients with lymphoma. Blood 47:211

Janka GE, Lau BM, Haas RJ (1978) Combination of chemotherapy and radiotherapy for Hodgkin's disease in children. Eur J Pediatr 127:282

Kögelmeier R (1982) Postsplenektomie-Infektionen und Pneumokokkenimpfung. Dissertation, University of München, München

Lanzowsky PH, Karayalcin G, et al (1975) Complications of laparotomy and splenectomy in the staging of Hodgkin's disease in children. Pediatr Res 9:389

Mufson MA (1981) Pneumococcal infections. JAMA 246:1942

Schellong G, Waubke AK, Langermann HJ, Breu H, Kuhne B, Riehm H, Ritter J (1982) Bedeutung klinischer und intraoperativer Befunde für die Voraussage eines Milzbefalls beim Morbus Hodgkin im Kindesalter: Eine retrospektive statistische Analyse bei 154 Patienten der Therapiestudie HD 78. Klin Pädiatr 194:242

Experimental and Clinical Experience with the Different Possibilities of Preserving Splenic Tissue After Rupture of the Spleen

M. Feldmann and M. Naber[1]

Today every surgeon or pediatric surgeon, when confronted with a splenic injury, must feel challenged to preserve the spleen by his therapeutic measures.

Apart from conservative observation, which waits for spontaneous healing under endoscopy and clinical intensive care, there are two basic methods at our disposal to preserve the entire spleen, parts of it, or at least some splenic tissue:

1. The preservation of the spleen or large parts of it in their topographical site (fibrin glueing, spleen suture, or partial resection)
2. Splenectomy followed by replantation of the splenic tissue in the form of splenic pulp, preferably into the greater omentum.

The second procedure is regarded as especially elegant because it imitates and partly intensifies the spontaneous tendencies of the organism, the so-called splenosis. The procedure enjoys increasing popularity among general surgeons and traumatologists because of ideal hemostasis and assumed protection against infection and postsplenectomy sepsis.

An absolute protection against postsplenectomy sepsis has not been proved either by means of animal experiments or from the few available clinical observations.

A few cases of fatal sepsis in the presence of intact spleen particles led to doubts about the effectiveness of this procedure (Holschneider et al. 1982).

Results of Our Animal Experiments

Three groups, each consisting of ten rats, were exposed to experimental peritonitis by inoculation with a suspension of rat feces. The animals in group 1 had a laparotomy only; group 2 had an additional splenectomy. In group 3 the whole spleen was reimplanted partly into the omentum, partly into the splenic lodge.

All experimental animals succumbed to the peritonitis. The mean survival time of the animals in group 1 was 5 days. The survival periods of group 2 and 3 were similar: all these animals died after 3 days.

[1] Chirurgische Klinik, Städt. Krankenanstalten Winterberg, D-6600 Saarbrücken/F.R.G.

Progress in Pediatric Surgery, Vol. 18
Ed. by P. Wurnig

Clinical Observations

From 1978 to 1983, 64 patients with spleen injuries were treated at the Winterberg Surgical Clinic in Saarbrücken. A quarter of these patients were less than 15 years old. Until 1980, in case of rupture of the spleen a splenectomy was carried out. Since 1981, we have been more concerned about the preservation of the spleen. Thus, in the years 1978–1980 there were 36 splenectomies, compared with only 12 splenectomies and 16 preserved organs in 1981–1982. The specific procedures and their problems are shown individually in Table 1.

From an examination of 100 spleens removed during earlier years, we found the most common injuries to be a torn parenchyma and multiple ruptures. Nowadays our operative procedure depends mainly upon the type of injury (Table 2). We have found out that only about one-fifth of the injured spleens cannot be preserved, so that reimplantation after splenectomy is indicated. Special circumstances, such as surgery on a patient with multiple trauma and shock, are not taken into consideration here; similarly the personal attitude of the surgeon towards preservation of the spleen is also not taken into account.

Table 1. Results and problems in operations in splenic injury (64 ruptured spleens 1978–1982)

	Fibrin glueing	Partial resection	Trans-plantation	Splenectomy
Postoperative bleeding	0/10	0/4	0/2	1/48
(literature)	0			3.7% (2)
Operative time	15–20 min	20 min	20–25 min	10 min
Septic complications (our experience)	0	0	0	4/48
Postsplenectomy sepsis (literature)	0	0	No certain protection	1%–2%
Unsolved problems	Risk of hepatitis		Later splenectomy (Hodgkin's disease)	Malignancy in asplenic organism

Table 2. The type of lesion indicates the choice of procedure

Lesion of capsule only	6%	Fibrin glueing with collagen fleece
Single rupture of parenchyma	40%	Fibrin glueing with or without collagen fleece
Abruption of one pole	12%	Partial resection;
Multiple rupture	21%	fibrin glueing with capsule or collagen fleece
Completely destroyed organ	9%	Splenectomy *and* transplantation
Disruption of artery	12%	

Discussion

Splenectomy is still considered to be the certain way to stop bleeding by many surgeons (Eraklis and Filler 1972). Thus, it can be understood that the replantation of splenic tissue after splenectomy is more widely practiced than the organ-preserving procedures of fibrin glueing and partial resection of the spleen.

Since protection against infection, especially against pneumococcal post-splenectomy sepsis, has so far been found only in the presence of intact spleens or intact spleen parts, splenectomy (followed by reimplantation of splenic tissue) should only be carried out if the spleen cannot be preserved by other methods (Cohen and Ferrante 1982).

Further experiments must prove whether a different technique of replantation will improve the protection against infections. In recent years, pediatric surgeons have often demanded to preserve the spleen using all available methods in spleen injuries, especially in infants and small children.

In our opinion this limitation to childhood is unjustified: every spleen, even in adults, is worth preserving.

Several reports give evidence that postsplenectomy sepsis in adults does occur.

It is a fact that most children with injured spleens are not treated by surgeons in a pediatric surgical center, but by general surgeons and traumatologists in small surgical departments.

In this case, only a surgeon with experience in operative preservation of the spleen in adults will also be prepared to carry out this procedure in children.

Summary

From clinical observation in adults, it is obvious that the preservation of the ruptured spleen is only possible in about 80% of all cases. Current evidence indicates that only the completely or partially intact spleen protects against pneumococcal sepsis. The best method of reimplantation has not yet been found.

Résumé

L'expérience clinique a prouvé que chez l'adulte, il était possible de conserver la rate lésée dans 4 cas sur 5. Seule une rate complète ou, les cas échéant, une rate partielle, assure la protection de l'individu contre la septicémie pneumococcique. Reste à trouver la meilleure technique de réimplantation de la rate.

Zusammenfassung

Klinische Erfahrungen beim Erwachsenen zeigen, daß die Erhaltung der rupturierten Milz in 4/5 der Fälle möglich ist. Derzeit bietet nur eine ganz oder partiell intakte Milz Schutz gegen Pneumokokkensepsis. Die beste Methode der Replantation ist noch nicht gefunden.

References

Cohen RC, Ferrante A (1982) Immune dysfunction in the presence of residual splenic tissue. Arch Dis Child 57:523–527

Eraklis AJ, Filler RM (1972) Splenectomy in childhood: a review of 1413 cases. J Pediatr Surg 7(4):382–388

Holschneider AM, Däumling S, Strasser B, Belohradsky BH (1982) Erfahrungen mit der heterotopen Autotransplantation von Milzgewebe im Kindesalter. Z Kinderchir 35:145–152

Incidence of Serious Infections After Splenectomy in Childhood

H. KÖNIGSWIESER[1]

With the Cooperation of Brandeis, W. E.[2], Gharib, M.[3], Gdanietz, K.[4], Holschneider, A. M.[5], Jürgenssen, O. A.[6], Lohr, J.[7], Tischer, W.[8], Urban, Ch.[9], Wählby, L.[10], Wurnig, P.[11]

There is international agreement which confirms the serious risks to splenectomized patients because of overwhelming postsplenectomy infections (OPSI) and other serious infections. By analysis of reports of individual cases (Appelbaum et al. 1979; Grinblat and Gilboa 1975; King and Shumacker 1952; Orlando and Moore 1972; Passl et al. 1976; Stögmann and Paky 1980; Tan 1982) and of collections of larger numbers (50–500) of patients (Belohradsky et al. 1982; Ein et al. 1977; Ellis and Smith 1966; Eraklis et al. 1967; Holschneider et al. 1982; Wählby and Domellöf 1981; Wählby 1981; Wegelius 1982) and from a few publications, which collected figure of more than 500 patients (Eraklis and Filler 1972; Erickson et al. 1968; Köglmeier 1982; Walker 1976), it is recognized that there is an extremely high risk of fatal infection following splenectomy.

The opinions regarding the extent of risk following surgery, as well as the nature of the disease, age of patient, and interval of time following surgery, vary widely. Only 2 or 3 years of age, the immediate postoperative period and certain operative indications were regarded as increasing the risk. Opinions about protective measures (pneumococcal vaccination and antibiotic prophylaxis) were also divergent (Balfanz et al. 1976; Diamond 1969; Passl et al. 1976; Platt 1982; Wegelius 1982).

Therefore we have tried to estimate the risk of OPSI in the central European area by means of collected statistics, which are discussed together, and to establish contemporary overview developed from previous experience and thus to clarify further questions.

At the 12th International Symposium of the Austrian Society of Pediatric Surgeons in January 1983, material on splenectomized patients was collected and the results were discussed. The results of this symposium will be presented here.

[1]Mautner Markhofsches Kinderspital der Stadt Wien, Baumgasse 35, A-1010 Wien/Austria
[2]Brandeis, W. E., Kinderklinik Heidelberg, Sektion Onkologie-Immunologie
[3]Gharib, M., Krankenanstalten der Stadt Köln, Kinderchir. Klinik
[4]Gdanietz, K., Noak, L., Städt. Klinikum Berlin-Buch, Kinderchirurg. Klinik
[5]Holschneider, A. M., Kinderchirurg. Klinik München
[6]Jürgenssen, O. A., Gherardini, R., Univ. Kinderklinik Wien u. II. Chirurg. Univ. Klinik Wien
[7]Lohr, J., Klotter, J., Hofmann v. Kap-herr, S., Pieper, W. M., Kinderchirurg. Univ. Klinik Mainz
[8]Tischer, W., Chir. Univ. Klinik u. Poliklinik, Kinderchirurg. Abt., Greifswald
[9]Urban, Ch., Muntean, K., Univ. Kinderklinik Graz
[10]Wählby, L., Enger, E., Henrikson, B., Univ. Hospital Umea, Dep. f. Chirurgie und Östra Sjukhuset Göteborg, Kinderchir. Klinik
[11]Wurnig, P., Ernstbrunner, Th., Mautner Markhofsches Kinderspital der Stadt Wien

Progress in Pediatric Surgery, Vol. 18
Ed. by P. Wurnig

Table 1. Survey of splenectomized patients

	Trauma	Benign hemato-logical diseases	Malig-nant hemato-logical diseases	Others	Total
FRG					
1. Brandeis	46	21	19	3	89
2. Gharib	19	22	1	3	45
3. Holschneider	19	72	25	34	150
4. Lohr et al.	42	–	–	–	42
GDR					
5. Gdanietz et al.	9	39	–	9	57
6. Tischer	6	13	11	1	31
Austria					
7. Jürgenssen et al.	–	12	13	3	28
8. Königswieser et al.	11	11	6	2	30
9. Urban et al.	–	32	9	1	42
Sweden					
10. Wählby et al.	413	92	9	11	525
Total	565	314	93	67	1039

The participants came from four European countries and were surveying a total of 1039 cases of splenectomized children (Table 1) over the last 15 years: 326 from FRG, 88 from GDR, 525 from Sweden, and 100 from Austria. The significant facts are presented in Tables 2, 3, and 4. From Table 1 it can immediately be derived that the combination of indications for splenectomy differs considerably. For some authors (Wählby and Domellöf 1981), the majority of splenectomies were done for spleen injuries, while other authors, e.g., Jürgenssen and Urban performed most of the splenectomies for hematological or oncological diseases. These facts must be considered in the evaluation of infection rate. Out of a total of 1039 cases collected in these statistics, 565 splenectomies were done for removal of an injured spleen, 314 for benign hematological diseases, 93 for malignancies, and 67 for other indications.

In Table 2 the relation between the indications for operation (i.e., the basic disease which required splenectomy) and the frequency and lethality of serious infections is presented. The four groups are the same as in Table 1. The largest included splenectomies for splenic injuries. The average age of the children in this group was 8.6 years at the time of operation. The group with benign hematological diseases requiring splenectomy included cases of microspherocytosis, idiopathic thrombozytopenic purpura (ITP), and so-called hypersplenism.

Table 2. Different indications for splenectomy and relation to severe postoperative infection and lethality

Indication	Patients (n)	Infections		Deaths		Overall lethality (%)
		n	(%)	*n*	(%)	
Trauma	565	30	5.3	5	16.6	0.9
Benign hematological disease	314	26	8.3	4	15.4	1.3
Malignant hematological diseases	93	22	23.6	8	36.4	8.6
Others	67	13	19.4	3	23.0	4.5
Total	1039	91	8.8	20	22.0	1.9

Splenectomies for malignant hematological diseases included Hodgkin's disease, leukoses, and cases of panmyelopathy, although the latter sometimes turned out to be advanced leukoses and the resistance against infection was typical for malignant diseases.

The average age of the patients with malignant hematological diseases was 10.6 years, while that of the children with benign hematological diseases was significantly lower at 8.2 years.

The group with other indications for splenectomy consisted of portal hypertension, thesaurismosis, and splenic cysts, among other diseases.

In accordance with statements in the literature (Dickerman 1979; Ein et al. 1977; Ellis and Smith 1966; Eraklis et al. 1967; Erickson et al. 1968; Walker 1976) the frequency of critical infections was lowest (5.3%) in the group of splenic injuries and somewhat higher in benign hematological diseases. It was by far highest in the patients with malignant hematological diseases (23.6%). Although serious infections appeared in the traumatic group less frequently than in benign hematological diseases, lethality was nearly the same in both groups. In contrast, in the malignant diseases it was more than twice as high at 36%.

In splenectomies for other indications infection rate was 19.4% and lethality 23% – also considerably higher than in the first two groups. Overall lethality from infection varied between 8.6% in malignant hematological diseases and 0.9% in traumatically caused loss of the spleen. It was 4.5% in the group with other indications. In the total of 1039 cases the rate of infection was 8.8%, 22% of which were lethal, so that an overall lethality rate of about 2% resulted.

If the cases of sepsis were separated from other serious infections, sepsis contributed 46 times (50.5%) to the total of 91 infection cases (Table 3).

In 18 of these cases (39%), *Streptococcus pneumoniae* was found. Two of the children suffering from sepsis had been vaccinated against pneumococcus and 11 had received antibiotic prophylaxis.

The comparison of serious infections in relation to the age of the children at time of operation (Table 3) shows that the frequency of severe infections was 53.6% in children under 36 mon, and three out of 15 died (20%). With increasing age, the rate of infection decreased.

Table 3. Severe infections and lethality related to the age of patients at time of splenectomy

Age	Patients (*n*)	Infections		Deaths		Overall lethality (%)
		n	(%)	*n*	(%)	
0–36 mon	28	15	53.6	3	20.0	10.7
37–72 mon	78	10	12.8	3	30.0	3.8
>72 mon	745	27	3.6	11	40.7	1.5
Total	851[a]	52	6.1	17	32.7	2.0

[a] 188 cases of Brandeis, Lohr et al., and Gdanietz et al. excluded

Table 4. Severe infections and time of appearance after splenectomy

Time interval	Infections		Deaths	
	n	%	*n*	%
0–36 mon	37	68.5	12	32.4
37–72 mon	13	24.1	5	38.5
>72 mon	4	7.4	0	0
Total	54	100.0	17	31.5

The rate of deaths, however, increased with increasing age: sepsis, therefore, does not decrease with increasing age. This increase in deaths could be attributed to the fact that children with malignant diseases were older and their chances of surviving sepsis must naturally be smaller. Therefore, it must be concluded that the danger caused by sepsis does not become slighter in children who are older at the time of operation, but that only the probability that a sepsis will occur is less.

Looking at the interval between operation and the appearance of severe infections (Table 4), it can be clearly seen that rate of death in cases of sepsis was rather constant in the first 6 postoperative years, whereas the frequency of infection in the first 3 years was nearly twice as high (68%) as in the 3- to 6-year-postoperative period. Six or more years after the operation the frequency of infection decreased significantly but was still present. It should be noted that in the cases where infections occurred more than 6 years after splenectomy, no deaths were recorded. From our observations and those of others, however, we can confirm that these infections were nevertheless of very critical character. Furthermore, we must remark that the average length of observation was 6 years, so that a final statement on infection frequency beyond 6 years cannot be made by us. Therefore, it will be necessary to continue further observations.

Many laboratory results were given in this material (blood count, thrombocyte count, immunoglobulins, complement level, etc.), which were obtained from postoperative examinations. They were, however, normal in most instances. It is therefore no need to mention them in detail.

Discussion

It became clear from the presented and discussed material that under present conditions in central Europe, splenectomized children are endangered by serious infections and sepsis. The risk of infection following splenectomy for ruptured spleen is 5.3%, after splenectomy for benign hematological diseases 8.3%, in cases with malignant hematological diseases 23.6%, and the death rate of manifest infections is between 15.4% and 36%.

Infection frequency in relation to underlying diseases corresponded to figures of other statistics already published (Belohradsky et al. 1982; Diamond 1969; Eraklis et al. 1967) but was three to five times as high as in the statistics of Gotoff (1973). (The percentages, however, concerned the incidence in individual groups.) Especially in malignant diseases, the incidence of sepsis seemed to be very high. This could be the reason why splenectomy for the purpose of staging, which was recommended during the last few years, is declining again today.

The significantly greater endangering of small children by OPSI is evident from our presentation, as is the prominent role of pneumococcal infections in 39%, even though they seem to be fewer than in other statistics, where they account sometimes for 50% (Belohradsky et al. 1982). Meningococcal infections, hemophilus infections, and staphylococcal infections were also observed.

The sepsis risk to the normal population in a highly civilized region like central Europe is surpassed three- to fourfold (Wählby and Domellöf 1981).

More than two-thirds of all recorded serious infections occurred in the first 3 postoperative years and most of the remaining third in the second 3-year period, but in individual cases there were serious infections even later.

No statement can be made from the material presented about the origin of such time differences in the incidence of infections.

Lethality following postsplenectomy infections is still considerable to be the greatest in malignant hematological diseases and is not necessarily lower in older children than in younger ones. This emphasizes the danger of this complication. A possible explanation for this observation would be that in the group of older children more malignant diseases are found, while in the younger group the splenectomies for spleen rupture dominate. On the success of prophylactic measures such as vaccination against pneumococci and antibiotic medication, no valid statement can be made from the presented material, since these measures were not consistently applied. It can be seen, however, that neither vaccination nor antibiotic prophylaxis provide absolute protection against severe infections, as several observations on our patients have shown.

The loss of two important functions of the spleen is responsible for the clinical affects of splenectomy. First, the cessation of the filter function and clearance of bacteria (Ellis and Smith 1966) and second, the lack of opsonins and a leucophile gamma globulin, or tuftsin, lead to a phagocytosis defect of macrophages and leucocytes, from which the capsule-carrying bacteria profit (Balfanz et al. 1976).

As a consequence of the high risk of sepsis in splenectomized children the following is necessary:

The spleen should be preserved as long as possible in elective splenectomies for hematological indications and in the case of splenic trauma, if it is at all possible. Only 25 g of splenic tissue – approximately one-sixth of the splenic mass of an older child – should suffice to maintain an adequate antibacterial splenic function (Eraklis et al. 1967). In the case of splenic trauma, modern diagnostic procedures (e.g., sonography) and therapeutic methods (fibrin glueing) allow organ-preserving treatment not possible in former times. Promising developments are on the way in the field of autotransplantation of splenic tissue.

Vaccination against pneumococci should be given because pneumococci account for a large number of infections, even though the presently available vaccine immunizes against only 14 capsule antigen types. The optimal effect of the vaccine is obtained when it is given at least 7 days before splenectomy. The development of the vaccine protection is disturbed in children under 2 years and those with suppressed immunity.

Antibiotic prophylaxis can be recommended in principle, whereby according to our results, it should be given for a minimum period of 3 years. Prophylaxis for 6 years is desirable and a longer period could possibly be indicated. Penicillin is an effective antibiotic for long-term prophylaxis – although not in every case (Appelbaum et al. 1977; Gumison et al. 1968; Jacobs et al. 1978) – against pneumococci and also meningococci. It can be given either continuously per os or as an intramuscular injection in monthly intervals. If fever occurs a broad spectrum antibiotic should be given as well; amoxicillin is especially recommended. Also after the termination of the long-term prophylaxis infections accompanied by fever should be immediately treated with antibiotics.

It is of special importance to explain the disease and treatment thoroughly to the patient's family and family doctor, to ensure maximum cooperation for prophylaxis and also for prompt treatment if infectious complications should occur. Apart from clinical observation over many years, up-to-date laboratory tests are not of decisive importance.

Summary

Ten groups of authors investigated their cases of splenectomized children in four different indication groups for frequency of postsplenectomy infection. Only severe infections were included and defined. A total of 1039 splenectomized patients were evaluated for the rate of infection and lethality following splenectomy. It was seen that in all groups there was a definite rate of infection and resultant deaths which was lowest in traumatic splenectomies and highest in malignant hematological diseases. The frequency of infection was highest in the early postoperative phase. Infections, however, still occurred more than 6 years after splenectomy. In older children the vulnerability to infection was less than in younger ones, but the mortality in older children was higher. The gravity of this danger can be seen, and effective therapeutic measures must be found and carried out. Especially, the attitude towards splenectomies should be changed in favor of spleen-preserving surgical procedures.

Résumé

Dans le but de préciser la fréquence des infections après splénectomie, 10 groupes d'auteurs ont étudié leurs enfants splénectomisés et les ont répartis en 4 groupes d'après l'indication. Seules les infections graves ont été retenues. La fréquence des infections et le décès éventuel consécutif ont été étudiés dans 1039 cas. Dans chacun des groupes, on a constaté un certain taux d'infection et de décès consécutifs. Le taux le plus bas était dans le groupe des splénectomisés traumatiques et le plus élevé dans celui des maladies hématologiques malignes. C'est pendant la phase post-opératoire que la fréquence des infections était la plus élevée, bien que des infections puissent se produire jusqu'à 6 ans après la spénectomie. Les grands enfants étaient moins sujets à une infection que les plus jeunes mais la mortalité était plus élevée chez les plus grands. Il s'agit donc d'un risque considérable et la définition et la mise en application de mesures thérapeutiques efficaces s'imposent. Chaque fois que cela est possible, il faut donner une préférence absolue à la conservation de la rate et renoncer à la splénectomie encore tant pratiquée.

Zusammenfassung

Zehn Autorengruppen untersuchten ihr Krankengut – aufgeteilt in 4 verschiedene Indikationsgruppen – auf die Häufigkeit von Postsplenektomieinfektionen hin. Nur schwere Infektionen wurden einbezogen und definiert. Infektionshäufigkeit und Letalität nach Splenektomie konnten bei insgesamt 1039 splenektomierten Kindern ausgewertet werden. In allen Gruppen konnte eine bestimmte Infektions- und Letalitätsrate aufgezeigt werden, die jedoch in der Gruppe der traumatischen Splenektomien am niedrigsten und bei den malignen hämatologischen Erkrankungen am höchsten war. Die Infektionshäufigkeit war am höchsten in der frühen postoperativen Phase; Infektionen traten jedoch noch mehr als 6 Jahre nach Splenektomie auf. Bei den älteren Kindern war die Infektanfälligkeit geringer als bei jüngeren, die Letalität jedoch höher. Daraus kann man die Schwere der Gefährdung durch diese Komplikation ersehen, die die Entwicklung effektiver Therapiemodelle erforderlich macht. Insbesondere sollte die noch durchgeführte Splenektomie durch organerhaltende Verfahren ersetzt werden.

References

Appelbaum PC, Scragg JN, Bowen AJ, et al (1977) *Streptococcus pneumoniae* resistant to penicillin and chloramphenicol. Lancet 2:995

Appelbaum PC, Shaikh BS, Widome MD, Gordon RA (1979) Fatal pneumococcal bacterimia in a vaccinated child. N Engl J Med 300:203

Balfanz JR, Nesbit ME Jr, Jarvis C, Krivit W (1976) Overwhelming sepsis following splenectomy for trauma. J Pediatr 88:458–460

Belohradsky BH, Däumling S, Roos R, Holschneider AM, Griscelli C (1982) Postsplenektomie-Infektionen und Pneumokokkenimpfung im kinderchirurgischen Bereich. Z Kinderchir 35: 140–144

Constantinopoulos A, Najar VA, Wish B (1973) Defective phagocytosis due to tuftsin deficiency in splenectomized subjects. Am J Dis Child 125:663

Diamond LK (1969) Splenectomy in childhood and the hazard of overwhelming infection. Pediatrics 43:886–889

Dickerman JD (1979) Splenectomy and sepsis: a warning. Pediatrics 63:938–939

Ein SH, Shandling B, Simpson JS, Stephens CA, Bandi SK, Biggar WD, Freedman MH (1977) The morbidity and mortality of splenectomy in childhood. Ann Surg 185:307–310

Ellis EF, Smith RT (1966) The role of the spleen in immunity. Pediatrics 37:111–119

Eraklis AJ, Filler RM (1972) Splenectomy in childhood: a review of 1413 cases. J Pediatr Surg 7:382

Eraklis AJ, Kevy SV, Diamond LK, Gross RE (1967) Hazard of overwhelming infection after splenectomy in childhood. N Engl J Med 267:1225–1229

Erickson WO, Burgert EO, Lynn HB (1968) The hazard of infection following splenectomy in children. Am J Dis Child 116:1–12

Gotoff SP (1973) Acquired and transient immunodeficiency disorders. In: Stiehm ER, Fulginiti VA (eds) Immunologic disorders in infants and children. Saunders, Philadelphia

Grinblat J, Gilboa Y (1975) Overwhelming pneumococcal sepsis 25 years after splenectomy. Am J Sci 270:523

Gumison JB, Frather MA, Pelcher EA, Jawetz E (1968) Penicillin resistant variants of pneumococcus. Appl Microbiol 16:311

Holschneider AM, Kricz-Klimeck H, Strasser B, Däumling S, Belohradsky BH (1982) Komplikationen nach Splenektomie im Kindesalter. Z Kinderchir 35:130–139

Jacobs MR, Koornhof HJ, Robins-Browne RM, et al (1978) Emergence of multiple resistant pneumococci. N Engl J Med 299:735

King H, Shumacker H Jr (1952) Susceptibility to infection after splenectomy performed in infancy. Ann Surg 136:239–242

Köglmeier R (1982) Postsplenektomie-Infektionen und Pneumokokken-Impfung. Dissertation, University of München, München – quoted by Belohradsky et al (1982) and Gotoff (1973)

Orlando JC, Moore TC (1972) Splenectomy for trauma in childhood. Surg Gynecol Obstet 134:94–96

Passl R, Eibl M, Egkher E, Frisee H, Gaudernak T, Neugebauer G, Vecsei W (1976) Splenektomie im Kindesalter aus traumatischer Ursache und ihre Folgen. Wien Klin Wochenschr 88:585–588

Platt R (1982) Infection after splenectomy. JAMA 248:2316

Stögmann W, Paky F (1980) Postsplenektomiesepsis. Pädiatr Praxis 23:429

Tan KH (1982) Fulminating pneumococcus septicemia and meningitis in an adult twenty years after splenectomy for a ruptured spleen. Neth J Surg 34:222–224

Wählby L (1981) Complications after elective splenectomy in children. Z Kinderchir 34:56–60
Wählby L, Domellöf L (1981) Splenectomy after blunt abdominal trauma. Acta Chir Scand 147: 131–135
Walker W (1976) Splenectomy in childhood. A review in England and Wales, 1960–1964. Br J Surg 63:36–43
Wegelius R (1982) Infections after splenectomy. Lancet I:1240
Wehinger H (1980) Milz und Milzexstirpation. In: Bachmann KD, Ewerbeck H, Joppich G, Kleihauer E, Rossi E, Stalder GR (Hrsg) Pädiatrie in Praxis und Klinik, Vol 2. Fischer, Stuttgart; Thieme, Stuttgart

Problems in Spleen Autotransplantation: Comparative Study of Types of Implantation in Animal Experiments

H. Roth[1] and R. Waldherr[2]

Spleen-preserving operations, either for maintenance of the whole organ or for partial resection, have absolute priority over autotransplantation when suitably indicated. Experimental examinations have shown that after the completion of the nidation phase, partial function of the spleen is taken over by the implants. The rate of survival of the experimental animals after intravenous pneumococcal exposure was, however, decreased, compared with those with intact, repaired, or partially resected spleens (Alwmark et al. 1983).

The seeming surgical simplicity of autotransplantation should not be the reason to make this the method of choice to preserve the function of splenic tissue. Clinical case reports of lethal pneumococcal sepsis after splenectomy in spite of splenosis peritonei (Böhm and Wybitul 1980; Rice and James 1980) indicate that iatrogenic localized splenosis apparently does not exclude the endangering of the patient, especially in the phase of revascularization and regeneration of the implants. In this period of at least 12 weeks (Likhite 1978), an asplenic status must be assumed. Pneumococcal vaccination and antibiotic prophylaxis are imperative until definite functional parameters are shown.

In spite of these limitations autotransplantation can be justified if hemostasis can only be achieved by splenectomy.

Other indications will be added, e.g., technically compelling indications for splenectomy in certain shunt operations due to portal hypertension.

An optimized standardization of the operative procedure for replantation has not been developed so far.

The individual surgical centers still use (besides scalpel and scissors) simple kitchen instruments such as a potato grater and a fruit pulp press to homogenize the spleen.

Necessary Conditions for Implant Nidation

The critical weight of a particle seems to be about 100 mg, according to Tavassoli et al. (1973). Larger fragments usually become entirely necrotic and show no regeneration. Homogenized spleen with destroyed microarchitecture also does not regenerate. Preservation of the microarchitecture, according to Alwmark et al. (1983), is absolutely necessary for nidation and growth of the implant. Further

[1] Kinderchirurg. Abt. des Chirurg. Zentrums und
[2] Pathologisches Institut der Universität, Im Neuenheimer Feld 110, D-6900 Heidelberg

Progress in Pediatric Surgery, Vol. 18
Ed. by P. Wurnig

premises are the removal of the splenic capsule, which presents an obstacle to diffusion (Seufert et al. 1981), and the reimplantation of all the homogenized tissue. Revascularization and quantity of perfused organ particles play a decisive role in the filter function and clearance of bacteria.

Preferred Areas in Animal Experiments

The question of the optimal place of replantation is still controversial. The tissue seems to nidate everywhere ubiquitously. As early as 1936, Perla observed spleen implant regeneration and microscopic revascularization at the ear lobe of an albino rat using a transparent chamber. The localizations shown in Table 1 were preferred in animal experiments.

Table 1. Autotransplantation of the spleen: preferred areas in animal experiments

Subcutaneous	Diffuse intraperitoneal
Intramuscular	Mesentery
Intrahepatic	Sigmoid mesocolon
Retroperitoneal	Lesser omentum

The examinations were first carried out from the viewpoint of implant regeneration, the amount of tissue to be transplanted, and functional effectiveness. The significance of the mutual connections between liver and spleen in transplant surgery, the direct drainage of the transplant blood into the portal venous outlet area, was first mentioned in 1981 by Vega et al.

Our Animal Experiments

Although our own efforts were at first mainly concentrated on the preservation of the orthotopic spleen of parts of the spleen with preserved arterial organ perfusion, we have been doing animal experiments with the different possibilities of spleen autotransplantation since 1981.

In Wistar rats weighing 250–300 g, using 15 animals for each chosen method, the following operations were carried out after splenectomy, capsule removal, and crushing of tissue to a particle size of 1–2 mm^3 maximum (Fig. 1).

1. Transplantation into the greater omentum:

The tissue was spread over the omentum, which was then rolled up, and the pocket thus formed closed with catgut stitches.

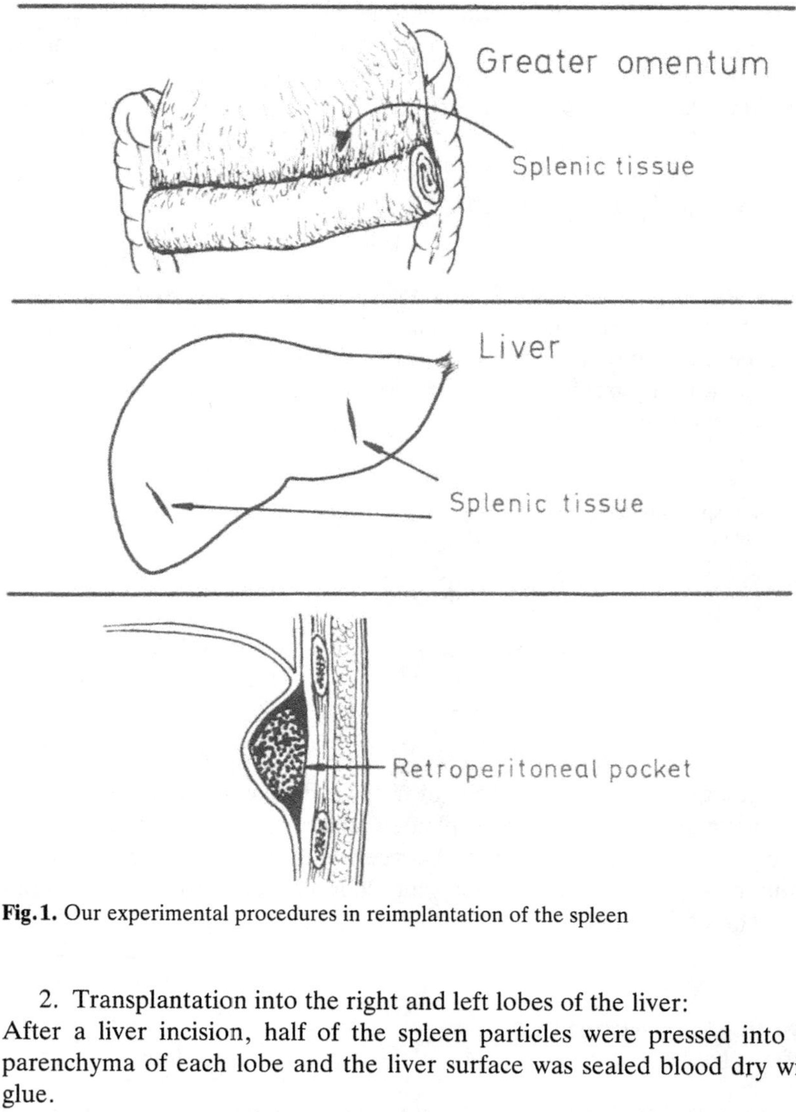

Fig. 1. Our experimental procedures in reimplantation of the spleen

2. Transplantation into the right and left lobes of the liver:
After a liver incision, half of the spleen particles were pressed into the liver parenchyma of each lobe and the liver surface was sealed blood dry with fibrin glue.

3. Retroperitoneal transplantation into a muscle pocket near the splenic bed in the upper left abdomen.

The animals were killed 6 weeks following surgery, and after macroscopic inspection, samples were taken from the transplantation site for microscopic examination.

Results

With transplants into the greater omentum, nidation of the implants in the omentum was confirmed as expected in nearly all cases. However, a tumorous pseudoabscess formation with tissue necrosis and a hard abscess membrane was found in three animals.

With transplantation into the liver, in all cases the transplantation site healed without complications and was covered by a scar of fibrous tissue. The result was histologically disappointing. In only five cases could splenic tissue be found. From the pathological viewpoint the fibrin glue seems to be a barrier to diffusion and nidation of tissue. According to Tavassoli et al. (1973) regeneration of the tissue particles starts after total necrosis of the margin areas. However, since the fibrin glue is replaced by less vascularized granulation tissue, this is possibly a plausible explanation for the lack of thriving of the implants, particularly because it is technically impossible to prevent an infiltration of the glue between the individual particles.

The retroperitoneal transplantation into a prepared muscle pocket gave no problems. In no case were there adhesions caused by the opening of the retroperitoneum. Splenic tissue could always be provid histologically.

Pathophysiological Aspects

Given these results, we have considered the following pathophysiological aspects. Implantation into the greater omentum is certainly a good method, where direct drainage into the portal venous system occurs. In animal experiments this has already been shown scintigraphically by Vega et al. (1981). Points of criticism are, however, the formation of pseudoabscesses and the possibility of acquiring infections or tumorous diseases involving the spleen. An example here is a case description by Gill (1944): the cause of a pseudoarthrosis of the tenth rib on the left side was scattered splenic tissue after rupture of the diaphragm and the spleen with a fracture of the tenth rib. During an attack of malaria, tumorous swelling developed in the area of the fracture. After resection of this "rib tumor," histologically vital splenic tissue was found.

The proximity to the intestinal tract and the pancreas and also the vulnerability of the omentum in children should be taken into consideration for a suitable site of transplantation. One must also keep in mind the preservation of access for later surgery or radiotherapy. Not only technical problems but also the possibilities of complications mentioned above exclude the liver as a site of implantation, although the criterion of functional unity between liver and spleen would be satisfied best. Autotransplantation into a retroperitoneal pocket near the splenic bed seems most likely to withstand all hesitations, with the exception of the demand for a direct flow of splenic venous blood into the portal venous system.

Our Alternative Procedure for Spleen Autotransplantation

It is known that the omentum in the form of a pediculated flap is often used in surgery for hemostasis in liver, spleen, and pancreas injuries or perforating injuries of the stomach and the duodenum. It is also used for blood supply of transplanted skin grafts at the abdominal and thoracic wall.

We see an alternative possibility to the surgical techniques currently in use in the following procedure:

After preparation of a pediculated omental flap, prepared spleen tissue (particle size maximum 1–2 mm^3) is spread over the omentum, the flap is rolled up (Fig. 2a), and the implant is positioned in a retroperitoneal pocket below the splenic bed with fixation stitches (Fig. 2b). The peritoneum is closed around the pedicle and the latter is fixed to the peritoneum.

Evident advantages are:

1. The good blood circulation of the greater omentum promotes the nidation of the transplants.
2. Connection with the portal venous system is provided.
3. The surgical and radiotherapy access is secured. Here silver clip marking within intraoperative plain abdominal X-ray film and later removal of the clips (to avoid scattering on computed tomography or echo shadows in sonographic examinations) can be helpful for localization of the implant.
4. The risk of bowel obstruction is largely excluded.

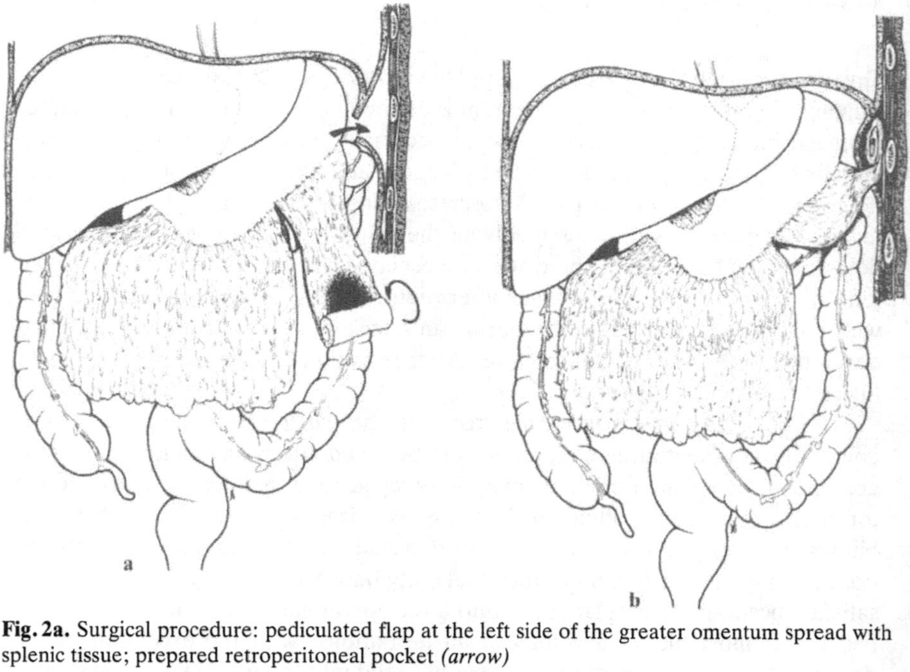

Fig. 2a. Surgical procedure: pediculated flap at the left side of the greater omentum spread with splenic tissue; prepared retroperitoneal pocket *(arrow)*

Fig. 2b. Retroperitoneally dislocated omental flap with splenic tissue

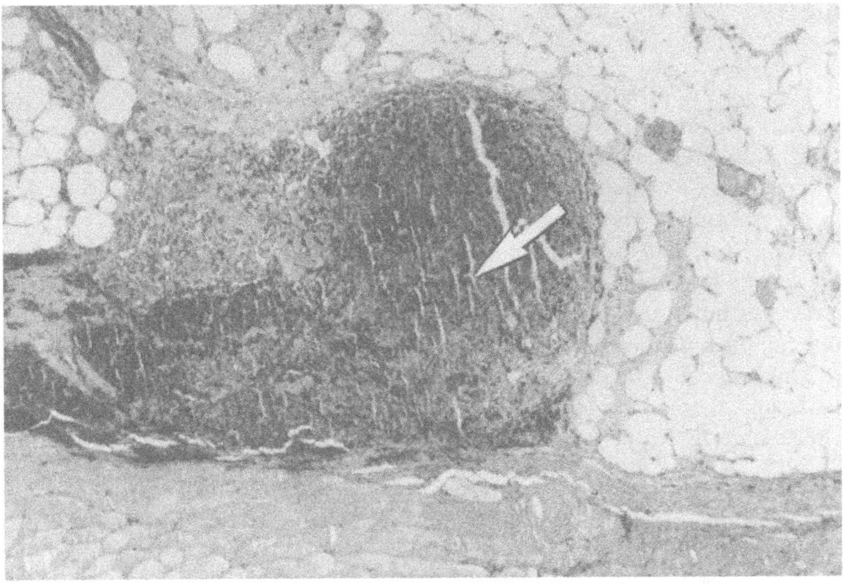

Fig. 3. 6 weeks after reimplantation. Vital splenic tissue between omentum and muscle pocket *(arrow)*

Our examinations in animal experiments with Wistar rats have been limited to anatomical factors so far. Both macroscopically and histologically, splenic tissue implanted in this way was identified as vital structure (Fig. 3). Scintigraphical and functional evidence is still lacking. Complete or partial autotransplantation of the spleen with dystope vessel connection is being tested experimentally at the moment.

Summary

Iatrogenic localized splenosis presents a seemingly simple surgical possibility for preserving partial function of the spleen. Until now, pathophysiological aspects, such as the drainage direction of venous blood from the spleen, possible splenic diseases in ectopic tissue, and the formation of pseudoabscesses as well as conditions for implantation have been given insufficient attention.

In 45 Wistar rats, divided into three groups according to the surgical procedure (implantation in the greater omentum, liver, retroperitoneum), the taking of the grafts were examined macroscopically and histologically. Because of the results, and bearing in mind the mentioned criteria, a new method for spleen autotransplantation is suggested: the implantation into a pediculated flap of omentum and retroperitoneal displacement behind the splenic bed.

Résumé

La splénose localisée iatrogène est une intervention en apparence très simple, destinée à sauvegarder partiellement certaines fonctions de la rate. Les aspects physiopathologiques: direction du drainage des veines spléniques, ectopie de tissue susceptibles d'être atteints, formation de pseudoabcès et nidation du transplant n'ont pas encore été suffisamment étudiés.

45 rats de l'Institut Wistar ont été partagés en 3 groupes, selon le genre d'intervention prévu: implantation dans le grand épiploon, le foie ou l'espace rétropérinéal et ces implantations ont fait l'objet d'une étude macroscopique et histologique. Sur la base des résultats obtenus et en fonction des critères cités au départ, on propose une nouvelle méthode de transplantation de la rate, soit l'implantation dans un fragment d'épiploon pédiculé avec mise en place rétropéritonéale dans le lit splénique.

Zusammenfassung

Die iatrogene lokalisierte Splenosis stellt eine chirurgisch scheinbar bestechend einfache Möglichkeit zur Erhaltung von Teilfunktionen der Milz dar. Pathophysiologische Gesichtspunkte wie Drainagerichtung des Milzvenenblutes, Ektopie potentieller Milzerkrankungen und Pseudoabzeßbildungen finden ebenso wie die Voraussetzungen zur Implantatnidation bisher nur ungenügende Beachtung.

An 45 Wistar-Ratten, aufgeteilt in 3 Gruppen entsprechend dem chirurgischen Vorgehen (Implantation: Omentum majus, Leber, Retroperitoneum), wurde makroskopisch und histologisch das Angehen der Implantate untersucht. Aufgrund der Ergebnisse und unter Berücksichtigung der obengenannten Kriterien wird eine neue Methode der Milzautotransplantation vorgeschlagen: die Implantation in einen gestielten Netzlappen mit retroperitonealer Verlagerung in das Milzbett.

References

Alwmark A, Bengmark S, Gullstrand P, et al (1983) Splenic resection or heterotopic transplantation of splenic tissue as alternatives to splenectomy. Regeneration and protective effect against pneumococcal septicaemia. Eur Surg Res 15:92

Böhm N, Wybitul K (1980) Autotransplantation von Milzgewebe nach traumatischer Milzruptur (traumatische Splenose). Chirurg 51:158

Gill AJ (1944) Traumatic autografts of splenic tissue in the body wall. J Lab Clin Med 29:247

Likhite VV (1978) Protection against fulminant sepsis in splenectomized mice by implantation of autochthonous splenic tissue. Exp Hematol 6:433

Perla D (1936) The regeneration of autoplastic transplants. Am J Pathol 12:665

Rice HM, James PD (1980) Ectopic splenic tissue failed to prevent fatal pneumococcal septicemia after splenectomy for trauma. Lancet 1:565

Seufert RM, Böttcher W, Munz D, et al (1981) Erste klinische Erfahrungen mit der heterotopen Autotransplantation der Milz. Chirurg 52:525

Tavassoli M, Ratzan J, Crosby W (1973) Studies on regeneration of heterotopic splenic autotransplants. Blood 41:701

Vega A, Howell C, Krasna I, et al (1981) Splenic autotransplantation: optimal functional factors. J Pediatr Surg 16:898

Subject Index